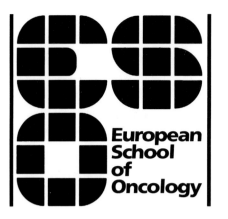

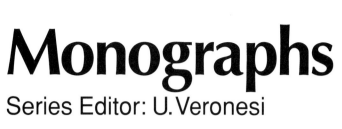

Series Editor: U. Veronesi

The European School of Oncology gratefully acknowledges sponsorship for
the Task Force received from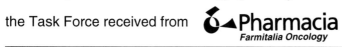

L. Denis (Ed.)

Prostate Cancer 2000

With 22 Figures and 30 Tables

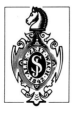
Springer-Verlag
Berlin   Heidelberg   New York
London   Paris   Tokyo
Hong Kong   Barcelona
Budapest

Chairman and editor:

Professor Dr. Louis Denis
Department of Urology
Algemeen Ziekenhuis Middelheim
Lindendreef 1
2020 Antwerp, Belgium

Co-chairman:

Professor G. P. Murphy
Chief Medical Officer
American Cancer Society
1599 Clifton Road N. E.
Atlanta, Georgia 30329, U.S.A.

ISBN 3-540-58296-7 Springer-Verlag Berlin Heidelberg New York
ISBN 0-387-58296-7 Springer-Verlag New York Berlin Heidelberg

Library of Congress Cataloging-in-Publication Data
Prostate cancer 2000 / L. Denis (ed.)
  (Monographs / European School of Oncology)
Includes bibliographical references.
  ISBN 3-540-58296-7 (alk. paper)
  ISBN 0-387-58296-7 (alk. paper)
1. Prostate--Cancer--Congresses. I. Denis, L. II. Title: Prostate cancer two thousand. III. Series: Monographs
(European School of Oncology) [DNLM: 1. Prostatic Neoplasms congresses. WJ 752 P9664 1994] RC280.P7P7423 1994
616.99'463--dc20 DNLM/DLC for Library of Congress

Typesetting: Camera ready by editor
Printing: Druckhaus Beltz, Hemsbach/Bergstraße;   Binding: J. Schäffer GmbH & Co. KG, Grünstadt
SPIN: 10087444   19/3130 - 5 4 3 2 1 0 — Printed on acid-free paper

Foreword

The European School of Oncology came into existence to respond to a need for information, education and training in the field of the diagnosis and treatment of cancer. There are two main reasons why such an initiative was considered necessary. Firstly, the teaching of oncology requires a rigorously multidisciplinary approach which is difficult for the Universities to put into practice since their system is mainly disciplinary orientated. Secondly, the rate of technological development that impinges on the diagnosis and treatment of cancer has been so rapid that it is not an easy task for medical faculties to adapt their curricula flexibly.

With its residential courses for organ pathologies and the seminars on new techniques (laser, monoclonal antibodies, imaging techniques etc.) or on the principal therapeutic controversies (conservative or mutilating surgery, primary or adjuvant chemotherapy, radiotherapy alone or integrated), it is the ambition of the European School of Oncology to fill a cultural and scientific gap and, thereby, create a bridge between the University and Industry and between these two and daily medical practice.

One of the more recent initiatives of ESO has been the institution of permanent study groups, also called task forces, where a limited number of leading experts are invited to meet once a year with the aim of defining the state of the art and possibly reaching a consensus on future developments in specific fields of oncology.

The ESO Monograph series was designed with the specific purpose of disseminating the results of these study group meetings, and providing concise and updated reviews of the topic discussed.

It was decided to keep the layout relatively simple, in order to restrict the costs and make the monographs available in the shortest possible time, thus overcoming a common problem in medical literature: that of the material being outdated even before publication.

Umberto Veronesi
Chairman Scientific Committee
European School of Oncology

Contents

Introduction

Louis Denis

Chairman International Prostate Health Council, Antwerp, Belgium

The symposium "Prostate Cancer 2000" was organised on the occasion of the tenth anniversary of the European School of Oncology. This monograph presents the contributions of the members of the E.S.O. Task Force on Prostate Cancer. The Task Force Programme of the School, supported by a Kabi Pharmacia grant, has resulted in the publication of two monographs on the "Medical Management of Prostate Cancer" in 1988 and 1990. This third monograph represents the major achievements in the field of prostate cancer in the USA and Europe, ranging from epidemiological concepts over treatment of localised disease towards new options in the treatment of hormone-independent cancer. Indeed, the timing of this symposium coincides with a great shift from treating metastatic disease towards curable localised disease by recent advances in early diagnosis and treatment, stimulating awareness and screening for prostate cancer. Great progress has been made by the U.S. National Prostate Cancer Program and the American Cancer Society, while the European Organisation for Research and Treatment of Cancer as well as the Europe Against Cancer Programme of the Community stimulated the development of new trials and the Pan European Screening Programme for Prostate Cancer.

It is my privilege to thank G.P. Murphy for his co-chairmanship of "Prostate Cancer 2000". We are indebted to the faculty for their enthusiam and dedication as well as their willingness to adapt their manuscripts after a joint discussion. We are grateful to Professor F. Pagano and Professor F. di Silverio for their guidance in the discussions of the symposium. We express our thanks for the extra educational support of Zeneca Pharmaceuticals and the International Prostate Health Council. The secretarial assistance of Mrs Rita Denie and the support of the responsible E.S.O. team, Carla de Jong, Vlatka Majstorovic and Director Alberto Costa, was vital to the completion of this monograph. The patience of Barbara Montenbruck of Springer Verlag is appreciated.

Prostate Cancer 2000: Projections for the Future

Gerald P. Murphy

Chief Medical Officer, American Cancer Society, 1599 Clifton Road N.E., Atlanta, Georgia 30329, U.S.A.

The detection and management of prostate cancer have improved considerably in the past decade and will be even more sharply defined in the future. Radiolabelled monoclonal antibodies are now available to detect occult soft tissue lesions of prostate cancer clinically by SPEC scanning. Lesions in lymph nodes and bone marrow are now visualised months before conventional techniques confirm this opportunity. As a result, the staging and earlier treatment of regionalised disease is possible.

Considerable efforts were made in the past for introducing chemotherapy and combined hormonal chemotherapy for more advanced disease, in the presence of widespread bony metastatic disease with little else to clinically evaluate. Smaller and earlier lesions of the prostate can be detected and confirmed by transrectal ultrasound and conventional markers such as prostate-specific antigen (PSA). PSA was originaly found to be helpful by the National Prostate Cancer Project in clinical trials. There are limitations, however. The screening of a healthy population is different from investigation of symptomatic individuals in an urologist's office. This issue, and its cost-effectiveness, will doubtless be resolved on a worldwide basis in the near future. Improvements in technology, be it by transrectal ultrasound or MRI or by other means, will considerably assist in this regard. For such a common tumour, it is remarkable that so little is known of the molecular origin of prostate cancer. The expression of a p21 protein product of the *ras* oncogene has been found to distinguish between carcinoma and benign hypertrophy. There are differential expressions of oncogene in cell culture, in response to a variety of hormonal milieus. More investigation is needed both in this field and into growth factors and their receptors in prostate cancer. Receptors for epidermal growth factor have been demonstrated and found to be higher in carcinoma than benign tissue. Tumour suppressor genes have also been implicated and there remain hopes for more correlation with other steroidal receptors.

These and other exciting developments may be able to contain the projected suffering and cost of prostate cancer in the 21st century. International collaboration will increase the efficacy of our efforts.

The Evolution of an Epidemic of Unknown Origin

Peter Boyle

Division of Epidemiology and Biostatistics, European Institute of Oncology, Via Ripamonti 332/10, 20141 Milan, Italy

It was estimated that there were six million cases of cancer diagnosed world-wide in 1980, of which 235,000 were cancer of the prostate [1]. In perspective, this compares with over half-a-million of each of stomach, lung, breast and large bowel and nearly 300,000 cancers of the oesophagus.

This gives a misleading impression of the numerical importance of prostate cancer which is characterised by large geographical variation in its incidence [2]. In the 12 member states of the European Community, it was estimated that in 1980 there were 85,000 new cases of prostate cancer, making it the second commonest form of cancer (after lung cancer) in men [3]. It has recently been reported that prostate cancer is the second most common form of cancer among men in the United States (after skin cancer) and is the second most common cause of death from cancer (after lung cancer). In 1992, an estimated 132,000 men in the United States will be diagnosed with prostate cancer and 34,000 men will die from this disease [4].

The situation in the United States at the present time has been evolving gradually. Between 1980 and 1988, age-adjusted incidence rates from prostate cancer increased among both black (Afro-American) men and white (caucasian) men, with the incidence rate higher in black men throughout the period of observation. The proportional increase in white men was a remarkable 30% which was considerably higher than the 8% increase observed in black men. Mortality rates also increased over this period, rising by 2.5% for white men and 5.7% for black men. Each year, the age-adjusted mortality rate was approximately double in black men compared to white men and there was also considerable variation in mortality rates between States. Among white men, mortality rates varied from 18.9 per 100,000 in Arkansas to 28.0 per 100,000 in Vermont: among black men, rates ranged from 29.8 per 100,000 in Minnesota to 55.5 per 100,000 in District of Columbia and North Carolina. It is notable that the highest rate in white men (Vermont, 28.0) was lower than the lowest rate recorded in black men (Minnesota, 29.8) [4].

Another way to assess the magnitude of the problem of prostate cancer is by considering the cumulative lifetime (up to age 75) risk. Based on 1985 age-specific incidence and mortality rates remaining unchanged throughout their lifetime, white men in the United States have an 8.7% lifetime risk of developing prostate cancer and black men a lifetime risk of 9.4 per cent. With regard to mortality from prostate cancer, the lifetime risks among whites and blacks in the United States are 2.6% and 4.3%, respectively.

Higher rates in black men than in white men, increases in overall trends in incidence and mortality rates and large geographical variations in occurrence are distinctive and recognised features of the descriptive epidemiology of prostate cancer [2]. Another feature of prostate cancer is the association between incidence (and mortality) rates and age, which is more striking than that for most other cancers. From an incidence rate of the order of 1-2 per 100,000 per annum in the forties the incidence rises dramatically to peak at 1,200 per 100,000 in white men and 1,600 per 100,000 in black men in their eighties.

This association with age has enormous consequences for the future. Assuming that age-specific incidence rates remain fixed at 1980 levels, the number of cases of prostate cancer in men aged over 65 in the European

Table 1. Cancer of the prostate in the European Community - Numbers of new cases in males aged 65+

Country	1990	2000	2010	2020
Belgium	2,796	3,156	3,248	3,939
Denmark	1,120	1,120	1,307	1,596
France	16,444	19,507	20,497	26,157
FR Germany	17,658	21,727	27,416	28,927
Greece	1,207	1,511	1,621	1,752
Ireland	549	546	621	814
Italy	11,321	13,510	14,836	16,313
Luxembourg	63	76	86	106
Netherlands	3,559	4,087	4,861	6,512
Portugal	1,753	1,993	2,068	2,347
Spain	8,056	9,938	10,454	11,933
United Kingdom	14,125	14,421	15,352	18,099
TOTAL EC	79,453	92,240	102,341	118,175
CANADA	6,494	7,784	9,391	12,927

Community will rise through 79,453 in 1990 to 92,240 in 2000. This increase in numbers of cases will be seen in every one of the 12 member states, being most pronounced in France, Germany and Spain (Table 1). The reason for this increase is that in these countries, as in most other countries, life expectancy is increasing: boys at birth can now expect to live to 80 years of age [5]. More and more men, living to older ages, will result in increases in the absolute number of cases of prostate cancer diagnosed even if the risk to an individual man remains fixed at 1980 levels.

This increase is programmed to continue into the 21st century and to be exacerbated in many countries. The post World War II "baby-boom" will be in their early fifties in the year 2000 and as they age will give rise to increasing numbers of cancers. This is the first group of men to go through life without the twin hazards of high infant mortality rates and a devastating war to contend with.

Looking around the world, the incidence of prostate cancer is increasing at an average annual rate of around 3% per annum. Some of this increase is undoubtedly associated with diagnostic artefact but the combined effect of this increase in incidence and the changing age structure of the population will be more pronounced for prostate cancer than for any other site in the majority of populations of the world. Again, assuming that the age-specific rates throughout the world remain fixed at their 1980 levels, the number of prostate cancers diagnosed throughout the world will increase from 235,000 in 1980 to 351,700 in 2000 if aging is the only contribution considered. If, however, this temporal trend continues, the result will be to increase the total burden to 492,000 new cases in the year 2000. It is clear that, even though the incidence rate may increase noticeably, the aging population will be the strongest determinant of the international prostate cancer burden in coming years.

These figures are perhaps underestimated: adding the European Community (1980) cases to those of the United States (in 1992) and the former USSR (in 1989) produces already a total of 228,000 cases. Advances in diagnostic technology during the 1980s have perhaps already resulted in these figures being biased downwards.

Beyond 2000, the numbers of cases of prostate cancer seem set to grow even quicker mainly due to the arrival of the post-World War II baby-boom to ages where prostate cancer will be a problem.

Prostate Cancer Control: 2000

The rise in the number of cases of prostate cancer requiring treatment will have important implications for the provision of treatment facilities including the training and supply of specialists competent to treat these patients. If it stopped here it would merely reflect an economic challenge but, unfortunately, increased numbers of cases will bring with it increased numbers of deaths from the disease. There are several complementary approaches to consider where means to reduce the mortality impact could be sought.

The best strategy from all perspectives would be the Epidemiology approach, i.e., to bring about a reduction in the incidence of prostate cancer through elimination and control of risk factors. Therapy also has a potentially important role to play since by improving the efficacy of treatment, increases in survival could be made which could contribute to an overall reduction in the mortality rate. Recently, the possibility of population screening for prostate cancer has attracted considerable attention: detecting prostate cancer at an earlier stage increases survival, but this has yet to be shown to be other than a lead-time bias.

Epidemiology

The ultimate aim of every epidemiological study is, through identification of determinants of disease risk, to delineate factors whose alteration would lead to individuals having less risk of disease and, consequently, lead to disease prevention. The best way, clearly, to reduce the mortality rate from a disease is to prevent the disease occurring.

Currently, two features of prostate cancer are well understood: it is a hormonally related disease and it may be avoidable.

Firstly, it is clear that the prostate gland is under hormonal regulation in that functional activity of the adult human prostate gland is largely dependent on plasma testosterone, of which over 90% of the daily production is synthesised and secreted by the Leydig cells of the testis. Within the prostate cell, testosterone is converted to 5-alpha Dihydrotestosterone (DHT) by the 5-alpha reductase enzyme system. DHT is essential for the growth and development of the prostate gland. Despite major increases in knowledge of our understanding of the endocrine and biochemical processes that regulate prostatic growth and function (see Griffiths in this volume), there is currently no consistent evidence of any primary endocrine disturbance that is necessarily implicated in the aetiology of prostatic cancer.

Secondly, the evidence that prostate cancer may be avoidable is compelling [6]. Briefly, different populations around the world experience different levels of prostate cancer and these levels change with time. Groups of migrants tend to acquire the prostate cancer pattern of their new homes within one or two generations of arrival: for example, Japanese migrants to the United States left behind the low levels of prostate cancer in Japan to adopt the higher levels of the local American population. Furthermore, population subgroups who share many common environmental factors but who have lifestyle characteristics which differentiate them from other members of the same community (e.g. blacks in US cities, Seventh Day Adventists, Mormons), have different levels of prostate cancer risk. For reasons such as these it is widely believed that prostatic cancer is a disease whose risk is determined by lifestyle or environmental factors and is, therefore, theoretically avoidable. Unfortunately, at the present time our knowledge of risk factors for prostate cancer is poor [2].

Therefore, despite many years of research it seems a remote possibility within our current knowledge of the aetiology of prostate cancer to define a successful strategy to reduce the risk of this disease based on findings from observational epidemiological studies.

The concept of chemoprevention of prostate cancer is attractive and there are a variety of agents which may be usefully considered at least on theoretical grounds. Retinoids, a term comprising vitamin A, beta-carotene and its derivatives, have been demonstrated to control differentiation and proliferation of various cell lines. However, the effects of dietary intake of vitamin A, carotene and retinol on prostate cancer risk have been inconclusive [7], with certain studies even suggesting prostate cancer risk increases with increasing vitamin A intake [6]. A recent experiment using Lobund-Wistar rats with prostate adenocarcinoma-III cells who were treated with 4-hydroxyphenol retinamide (4-HPR) demonstrated that metastatic disease was significantly reduced.

However, this experiment was small and a larger experiment is currently being completed in the laboratory of Michael Sporn at the National Cancer Institute in Bethesda, United States. The findings from this will have considerable influence on future possibilities for chemoprevention. They will need to be convincing to offset the persistent doubts of positive associations found in human epidemiological studies which, however, have been characterised by being of low quality. Furthermore, there is also the hurdle of toxicity to approach. In a long-term chemoprevention study, involving tens of thousands of men taking a compound for prolonged periods of time (up to 10 years), even minimal levels of toxicity could lead to significant compliance problems and make interpretation of findings problematic. 4-HPR has the unwanted side effects of dark adaptation and skin toxicities: in animal studies, chronic feeding of 4-HPR has been noted to cause body weight reduction and reduction in food intake as well as hepatomegaly and increases in SGPT, serum cholesterol and triglyceride levels.

The possible role of 5-alpha reductase inhibitors in chemoprevention of prostatic cancer is currently being assessed and debated. This is a new class of products designed initially for the treatment of benign prostatic hyperplasia. In the absence of DHT, the prostate will be expected to "shrink": the 5AR enzyme is necessary for the conversion of T(estosterone) to DHT and blocking this enzyme reduces DHT levels available to the prostate. The initial observation that male pseudohermaphrodites, who have an inherited 5AR deficiency, do not develop BPH or prostate cancer gave early motivation to consider the role of 5AR in prostate cancer chemoprevention. Its potential is confirmed by a number of other observations. The development of prostate cancer is influenced by the androgenic milieu of the prostate in some way, and so it seems immediately plausible that interfering with this milieu may alter disease risk. A recent study compared testosterone, sex hormone binding globulin (SHBG) and two indirect measures of 5AR activity in serum [3-alpha, 17 beta-androstanediol glucoronide (a-diol-g) and androsterone glucoronide (A-g)] levels in 50 United States caucasians and 50 blacks and 54 young Japanese men. Black men had 11% higher testosterone levels and 9% higher SHBG levels. Significantly higher levels of a-diol-g and A-g were detected in blacks and in whites than in Japanese [8]. These data are very indirect and cannot be interpreted in terms of causality but are consistent with reduced 5AR activity playing a protective role in the development of prostate cancer in Japanese men.

Five-alpha reductase inhibition has also been shown to cause dose-dependent inhibition of two human prostate cell lines *in vitro*.

Given that the development of prostate cancer is influenced by the androgenic milieu of the male, that inherited 5-alpha reductase deficiency prevents the development of the prostate and diseases of the gland, that population groups at different risk of prostate cancer may have different levels of 5AR activity, that one 5AR inhibits prostate cancer cells *in vitro* and that this product has a very low risk of side effects and a high compliance rate in clinical trials, then consideration should be given to taking steps to conduct trials of well-men to assess its potential. These steps range from more laboratory studies to more clinical research.

One problem with this strategy would be that with the ever-increasing use of PSA (prostate specific antigen) as a diagnostic test for prostate cancer, given that 5AR use is associated with up to 50% reductions of PSA, then there is a danger that early prostate cancers in the treatment group would be "masked" and/or more biopsies would be performed in the control group and, hence, more early tumours found.

Phase III studies of the 5 alpha reductase inhibitor have shown a very positive, low-side-effects profile. The only significant differences in side effects, comparing a group receiving 5 mg compared to the placebo group, were with reports of decreased libido (4.7% versus 1.3%) and ejaculatory disorder (4.4% versus 1.7), the latter a minor complication resulting from the physiological action of the compound. Only 2% withdrew because of side effects. However, while this is very acceptable in a clinical study of diseased, symptomatic individuals, it may reduce recruitment and compliance in normal men. There may be a need to consider whether an acceptable level of side effects in a clinical trial would necessarily be acceptable to a healthy group of men.

These and other problems should be addressed with some urgency since there is some promise in pursuing this direction although we are still at an early stage.

Therapy

The treatment of prostate cancer is discussed in various other chapters in this book, covering both surgical and hormonal approaches. In the opinion of this reviewer, improvements in the treatment of prostate cancer appear to be overdue. While there have been advances in surgical, radiotherapeutic and hormonal therapy, there is yet to be an important contribution from medical oncology.

This aspect deserves urgent attention given the increasing importance of prostate cancer as a Public Health priority. Rather than rooting around in the (bottom of the) barrel of traditional cytotoxic agents, medical oncologists should give both attention and intellectual innovation to the treatment of prostatic cancer.

Screening

Digital rectal examination (DRE) [9], prostate-specific antigen (PSA) [10] and transrectal ultrasound (TRUS) [11] have all been demonstrated as being capable of identifying tumours in the prostate at an early stage (i.e., pre-symptomatic) [12]. Although the technologies for conducting population screening may be available, at the present time there is not enough evidence to advocate the implementation of widespread prostate screening activities: the screening tests available, alone or in combination, have not yet been properly characterised in terms of their sensitivity and specificity and none have been satisfactorily demonstrated to lead to a "true" reduction of mortality from prostate cancer. However, the current situation goes a long way to meeting the criteria of Wilson and Jungner [13] to judge whether screening can be advocated at least on a trial basis [14].

The current situation of prostate screening (with DRE, PSA, TRUS) is strikingly similar to the situation in the mid-1960s when mammography began to become available for detecting breast cancers. Above all, there is a need to determine whether the existing favourable signs for prostate cancer will prove to be correct, with confirmation that mortality can be reduced by screening and a tension between those who appreciate the need for large, expensive studies that avoid biases and those who would prefer to use "simpler" although incorrect analyses (e.g. survival increases detected by screening). There is current concern regarding the possible costs of work-up for those men found positive on screening and the potential for "over-diagnosis" which is in many ways similar to the situation regarding breast cancer in the mid-1960s. The current situation regarding breast cancer, where national mammographic screening programmes are now being implemented in several countries, was based on 4 large randomised trials involving 280,000 women. The mortality reduction among women aged 50-64 years appears to be around 20% and this gives another clear message to those currently considering prostate cancer screening: trials must not only be large and randomised but a realistic estimate of mortality reduction must be made at the start (when sample size is being calculated). At least 5-8 years were "lost" in breast cancer because trials had been designed to detect a mortality reduction of 30% and needed larger follow-up to have power to detect the 20% reduction found.

The lessons learned from breast cancer screening with mammography, particularly with regard to study design, provide a vindication of the policy of evaluating screening through properly conducted randomised trials.

Randomised trials, however, will never be a panacea which provides all the answers required and current investigators should be reminded of the need for size both in numbers entered into the studies and the follow-up.

I see, however, exciting developments in prostate cancer with screening trials offering a real prospect of being successful and some prospects for chemoprevention. Much more information is urgently needed, particularly about risk factors, to help control the prostate cancer explosion which is programmed to occur.

Acknowledgements

It is a pleasure to acknowledge the contribution to my understanding of the epidemiology of prostate disease made by Professor L. Denis, Professor K. Griffiths, Professor F. Schroeder, other members of the International Prostate Health Council and Dr. Baudoin Standaert.

REFERENCES

1 Parkin DM, Laara E and Muir CS: Estimates of the worldwide frequency of sixteen major cancers in 1980. Int J Cancer 1988 (41):184-187

2 Zaridze DG and Boyle P: Cancer of the prostate: epidemiology and aetiology. Br J Urol 1987 (59):493-503

3 Jensen OM, Esteve J, Moller H and Renard H: Cancer in the European Community and its member states. Eur J Cancer 1990 (26):1167-1256

4 World Health Organisation: Trends in prostate cancer 1980-1988. WHO Weekly Epidemiological Record 1992 (67):281-288

5 Brody J: Prospects for an aging population. Nature 1985 (315):463-466

6 Boyle P: The epidemiology of prostate cancer. In: Denis L (ed) Recent Advances in the Medical Management of Prostate Cancer. Springer-Verlag, Heidelberg 1990

7 Mayne ST, Graham S and Zheng T: Dietary retinol: prevention or promotion of carcinogenesis in humans? Cancer Causes Control 1991 (2):443-450

8 Ross RK, Bernstein L, Loba RA, Shimizu H, Stanczyk FZ, Pike MC and Henderson BE: 5-alpha-reductase activity and risk of prostate cancer among Japanese and US white and black males. Lancet 1992 (339):887-889

9 Pedersen KV, Carlsson P, Varenhorst E et al: Screening for carcinoma of the prostate by digital rectal examinations in a randomly selected population. Br Med J 1990 (300):1041-1044

10 Catalona WJ, Smith DS, Ratliff RH et al: `Med 1991 (324):1156-1161

11 Waterhouse RL and Resnick MI: The use of transrectal prostatic ultrasonography in the evaluation of patients with prostatic carcinoma. J Urol 1989 (141):233-239

12 Bentvelsen FM and Schroeder FH: Modalities available for screening for prostate cancer. Eur J Cancer 1993 (29A):804-811

13 Wilson JMG and Jungner G: Principles and practice of screening for disease. Public Health Paper No 34, WHO, Geneva1969

14 Boyle P, Alexander FE, Standaert B and Denis L: Screening for prostate cancer. In: Hendry W and Kirby R (eds) Recent Advances in Urology. Churchill-Livingstone, Edinburgh 1993

Remarks on Screening and Early Detection of Prostate Cancer

Fritz H. Schröder

Department of Urology, Erasmus University and Academic Hospital, P.O. Box 1738, 3000 DR Rotterdam, The Netherlands

In order to justify screening for malignant disease of any type the tumour under consideration must be frequent. There must be an identifiable early stage and early treatment must be shown to have a favourable impact on quantity and quality of life of such patients. Screening for prostate cancer (PC) is an issue of great controversy at this moment. In some countries such as Germany governmental early detection programmes have been implemented. In some other countries such as The Netherlands and Britain early detection for this disease is not supported by the government and health insurance policies. As a result of the availability of more invasive screening tests, these are used in the general population with increasing frequency. Screening for prostate cancer and early detection have been subjects of extensive study and review recently [1-5]. It cannot be the purpose of this presentation to add another review. Practical and controversial aspects will be dealt in a simple and practice-oriented manner.

Incidence and Mortality of Prostate Cancer

Prostate cancer is the second most frequent malignancy in men in most European countries. The overall incidence of the countries of the European community during the years of 1978-1982 amounted to 54.9/100,000. This is equal to a life-time risk of 3.9% based on 75 years of life expectancy. Due to competing causes of death and the relatively slow rate of progression of locally confined disease, the age-corrected mortality amounts to only 22.6/100,000, i.e., a life-time mortality of 1.2% [6].

There is a strong geographic variation of prostate cancer. The incidence and the life-time risk in the United States are considerably higher than in most European countries. On the other hand, in other countries such as Japan, China and Singapore incidence and mortality are roughly 10-fold lower than in western European countries [7]. A good explanation for these differences is not available. The fact, however, that preclinical lesions found at autopsy are equally frequent in countries with a low or high incidence of clinical prostate cancer clearly points to a pathogenesis that can be divided into a phase of initiation and a second phase of promotion. Promotion is dependent on geographical and probably lifestyle factors.

Incidence and mortality have been rising in recent years in most countries with a high incidence. Part of this rise is due to increasing male longevity. However, there is also a true increase which is unexplained at this time. The fact that the ratio of mortality and incidence is not decreasing indicates that the increase in incidence is not due to more frequent diagnosis of very early stages [8].

Fifty to sixty percent of all cases of prostate cancer are diagnosed with distant metastases present and are beyond any chance of cure.

Latent versus Manifest Disease

Most carcinomas of the prostate are palpable at rectal examination. The fact alone that a simple, non-invasive technique is available to identify this disease seems to advocate early detection programmes. However, the story is more complicated.

Tigers and Pussycats ?

In autopsy series prostate cancer is found in about 30% of 50-year-old males. Most of these tumours are focal in nature. The chance of a 75-year-old man to present with such lesions at autopsy has been calculated to be 42% [4]. If one compares these figures with the European life-time risk of acquiring prostate cancer of 3.9%, a 10.8-fold difference results. Only 3.9 of 42 cancers will surface clinically during a life-time of 75 years. Obviously, if focal lesions as they are discovered at autopsy would be picked up clinically, overdiagnosis and overtreatment would result. It is obvious that differentiation between tigers and pussycats is mandatory.

Which Cancers Are Clinically Relevant ?

Unfortunately, at this moment there are no parameters available which conclusively allow to predict at the time of the diagnosis of locally confined disease which of these tumours will progress and which will remain "dormant". While it has been demonstrated that even very small tumours have a high rate of proliferation, as shown by means of double labeling techniques, and that the proportion of non-diploid tumours even in focal disease is similar to clinical disease, there is clear evidence that with the increase in size loss of differentiation occurs. To the best of present knowledge truly focal tumours are small, i.e., they have diameters of 1-2 mm amounting to volumes of 0.004 ml. Even if 2-3 such focal tumours are present in histological slides, the total volume would still only be in the range of 0.015 ml. The smallest detectable, non-palpable tumours at ultrasonography have diameters of 0.7 cm, resulting in a volume of approximately 0.2 ml [9]. Also, clinically relevant disease is usually not well differentiated, has an invasive pattern of growth and originates from the peripheral zone of the prostate. Scardino and co-workers [4] have convincingly shown that very small carcinomas are quite rarely diagnosed clinically and that cancers diagnosed by TURP, DRE and TRUS as well as by PSA-driven screening have average volumes of 3.93, 5.4, 4.19 and 7.12 ml, respectively. So there is increasing evidence that truly focal disease is only rarely diagnosed by routine clinical techniques except as incidental carcinoma at the time of surgery for benign disease. Roughly half of the incidentally found tumours belong to the focal group. Overall it is estimated that only about 4% of clinically identified cancer is truly focal in character.

So maybe the fear that the typical "autopsy cancers" are diagnosed is not well founded. Still, considerable controversy exists as to whether treatment for clinically identified localised disease is necessary, and, if applied, whether a substantial proportion of patients managed by radiotherapy or radical surgery can be cured of their disease with a resulting prolongation of their lifespan.

Natural History and Results of Treatment

Recent evidence seems to indicate that confined prostate cancer has a doubling time of about 2 years [10]. Carter et al. [11] show that even in the preclinical stage of prostate cancer an exponential rise of plasma levels of prostate-specific antigen (PSA) occurs which allows to calculate an average doubling time of 2.5 years. Clinically, according to the available information which has been summarised in [5], truly focal disease has a median time to either local or systemic progression of 13-15 years, while incidentally found non-focal disease progresses in a median time of 5 years. For palpable lesions which are locally confined progression rates varying between 35-78% have been described within observation times of 5-10 years. In the few surveillance studies which are available very few patients, however, die of prostate cancer. These data are used by those who are sceptical about early detection and screening to argue that the usefulness of treatment can only be shown in a randomised prospective study comparing aggressive treatment to a wait-and-see policy. Unfortunately, statistically solid and clinically relevant studies of this type are unavailable. Proponents of early detection and aggressive management argue that there is a very large discrepancy in 5 and 10-year survival rates between patients who are diagnosed and treated with metastatic disease and those who undergo potentially curative management for locally confined disease. While median survival time with metastatic disease and endocrine treatment is only in the range of 30 months, patients who are aggressively treated for palpable nodular disease within their prostate have an 80-85% 5-year survival and share the life expectancy of other age-matched men who do not suffer from prostate cancer. Also, it turns out that tumours identified with traditional diagnostic techniques dominated by rectal examination (DRE) are often too extensive for total excision or effective radiotherapy. Twenty-five percent of those who are thought to be resectable turn up with positive margins of resection. Another 25% will have evidence of lymph-node metastases at the time of surgery. Early detection programmes which combine prostate-specific antigen, rectal examination and ultrasonography are capable of detecting cancers which are more frequently confined to the prostate and with a low incidence of lymph-node metastases which is only in the range of 5-10% [12]. Unfortunately a clear advantage in survival or cancer mortality for patients who are treated aggressively is not evident from historical comparison of treatment and surveillance studies. Important prognostic factors which govern prostate cancer mortality are present in all these series and are difficult to correct for retrospectively.

How Much Overtreatment Can Be Expected in Early Detection Programmes?

In discussions of this problem very often the autopsy prevalence, cumulative or in certain age groups, which ranges from 15-100% is compared to annual incidence rates of prostate cancer. This comparison obviously is not correct because the life-time risk is not considered in incidence data while autopsy data represent more closely the cumulative life-time risk of attaining this disease. In Table 1 more comparable information is presented. The figure of 32.9% presents the cumulative prevalence in the study of Franks [13] for the ages of 50-90+. In the age group 70-79 in his study the prevalence was 40.0%. Franks studied 210 patients and found that most of the identified latent tumours were focal but 52 of the 69 cancers already seemed to be infiltrating the fibrous capsule of the prostate. In a similar study by Gaynor [16] which was published as early as 1938, 1050 patients were studied. The cumulative prevalence was 18.2%; obviously, autopsy prevalence among other factors depends on preparative techniques. The prevalence at age 70-79 was 67 of 237 patients, or 28.3%. As mentioned above, from all available literature data a life-time risk for a 75-year-old man of having prostate cancer at autopsy was calculated to be 42% [4].

Table 1. Cumulative incidence and risk of dying of prostate cancer

	Cancer found	Ratio*	Reference
Autopsy series	32.9%	27	[13]
EC clinical incidence	3.9%	3	[6]
Detection rate in population-based screening studies	2.5%	2	[1,14]
Prevalence incidental carcinoma	14.0%	11	[15]
EC cumulative mortality	1.2%	1	[6]

* Ratio = proportion of males not expected to be at risk of dying from PC

The cumulative incidence of prostate cancer for the European community was calculated to be 3.9% at age 75. The cumulative mortality over the same period is 1.2%. The detection rate in screening studies is in the range of 2.5%. Unfortunately this does not represent the lifetime risk of having prostate cancer detected with repeated application of early detection measures. Data on rescreening are inconclusive at the moment. Estimations of life-time risk in detection studies might be possible in the future as a result of prospective screening studies which will allow estimations of lead- and length-time bias as well as through estimations on the basis of the observation of an exponential rise of PSA values in men without clinical evidence of prostate cancer.

The ratios indicated in the second column of Table 1 indicate that in relation to every death from prostate cancer 3.3 carcinomas are diagnosed clinically, 11.7 incidental carcinomas are found, 2.1 cancers are detected at one-time screening and 27.4 cancers would be detected at autopsy series. The amount of overtreatment is likely to be within the range of these data. Based on the information that is available on rescreening at this moment, one can assume that the detection rate will at least be doubled as compared to DRE alone. On the other hand, if one uses current treatment policies and excludes truly focal disease identified as incidental carcinoma from treatment, the prevalence of incidental PC will be 7% instead of 14%. With these assumptions, countries and institutions that embark on population-based early detection programmes and decide to treat all patients identified by radiotherapy or radical prostatectomy, will have to accept overtreatment in the range of 4-7 times the risk of dying of the disease.

The Screening Tests

One of the prerequisites for applying screening for any disease to the general population is the availability of effective screening tests. Positive predictive values above 80% with a high specificity are desirable. None of the screening tests which are available for the detection of prostate cancer fulfils these requirements. The efficiency of rectal examination

Table 2. Sensitivity and positive predictive values for DRE, TRUS and PSA in the detection of prostate cancer

Screening test	Sensitivity	Positive predictive value
DRE	45-82%	28%
TRUS	60-91%	31%
PSA > 4 ng/ml	77%	24%
PSA > 10 ng/ml	43%	60%

The data are based on a review of studies which are population or urology clinic based [17]

(DRE), determinations of prostate-specific antigen (PSA) in plasma and transrectal ultrasonography (TRUS) have been reviewed recently by several authors including Bentvelsen et al. [17]. The data resulting from this rather complete literature review on sensitivity and positive predictive values are indicated in Table 2.

The question whether a combination of 2 or 3 of the screening tests will be sufficiently sensitive and specific for use in this disease is currently the subject of intensive investigation around the world. At this moment it appears that DRE and PSA as primary tests may be suitable and may also fulfil the requirement of being acceptable to the male population. One of the problems is a low specificity leading to a high proportion of false-positive rectal examinations and, because of the overlap with benign prostatic hyperplasia especially of larger volumes, also of PSA even above 10 ng/ml. Lesions that are suspicious on rectal examination and that are biopsied turn out to be cancerous in 40-50% of cases. The proportion of negative biopsies is considerably higher if the suspicion is based only on abnormal PSA values combined with an abnormal DRE or TRUS study. One of the lines of research that may lead to an improvement of the positive predictive value and the specificity of the screening studies is the correction of plasma PSA values with prostatic volume. Lee et al. [9] have shown that the positive predictive value for a TRUS-guided biopsy can be raised to 86% in a group of patients with BPH and non-palpable prostate cancer if only those plasma PSA

Table 3. Possible algorithm for early detection of prostate cancer by DRE, PSA and TRUS

DRE	PSA	Further diagnostic policy
Normal	≤ 4.0*	None
Normal	4.0 - 10.0 **	TRUS + biopsy of suspected lesions
Normal	> 10.0	TRUS + biopsy of suspected lesions
Abnormal	-------->	TRUS-guided biopsy

*   hybritech assay, ng/ml
** some correction of PSA for gland volume should be applied, in the future an indication for biopsy of non-suspicious prostates may result

values are considered that are above the regression line correlating BPH volume and plasma PSA values.

In Table 3 a possible algorithm for the use of early detection tests is presented. Considering the high risk (15-20%) of the presence of prostate cancer in patients with obstructive symptoms [2], this algorithm should certainly be applied to this group of patients. In the author's view, a broad use in the general population is not warranted at the moment.

If rectal examination and PSA are normal, which may be expected to be the case in about 85% of men, no further studies are recommended. If PSA values are in the range of 4.0-10.0 ng/ml, which is the case in 8-9% of the general population, the chance of harbouring detectable prostate cancer is about 25%. In this group TRUS and biopsy of suspicious lesions is recommended. In the future correction of plasma PSA values by gland volume in some form may lead to an indication for biopsy even in absence of suspicious lesions on rectal examination or ultrasonography. The same policies should be applied if rectal examination is normal and PSA values are above 10 ng/ml. The chance of finding prostate cancer in this group is around 60%, PSA above 10 ng/ml is found in 2-3% of the general male population above 50 years of age. In many European studies it has been shown that 20% of these elevated PSA values can be explained by the presence of BPH. Again, correction with gland volume may sharpen the indication for biopsy in the future. An abnormal rectal examination which is suspicious for prostate cancer should also be an indication for a biopsy.

Which Role Should Early Detection Tests Play in Current Clinical Practice?

In absence of conclusive data showing benefit in terms of cancer mortality or overall survival or even in terms of quality of life for patients whose prostate cancer is detected early and treated aggressively, various policies have been adopted in different countries. In Germany early detection of prostate cancer has been a public health policy since 1978. In Belgium a general health test which is paid for by insurance companies includes a rectal examination. The American Cancer Society and the American Urological Association have recommended an annual rectal examination and PSA determination for males above 50 years of age. A recent survey in the United States which included 4.7% of all urologist members of the American Urological Association has shown that the use of an annual rectal examination was unanimously recommended as a routine for the urological examination as well as for prostate cancer detection. Prostate-specific antigen was recommended by a majority of the respondents for both situations, the diagnostic workup with symptoms of prostatism and for routine use in early detection [18]. It seems that the scientific rationale for the use of these tests on the basis of clinical benefit, cost benefit and other objective parameters does not determine clinical practice. Males are worried about prostate cancer, they know about the availability of the tests, they do not care about the statistics involved but wish to get rid of cancer if diagnosed early and if at all possible. It is understandable that urologists and general medical practice yields to this demand. It is the policy of the author of this article to tell patients about the strong possibility of overdiagnosis and overtreatment and to offer surveillance rather than aggressive treatment in the first place. Still, most patients after careful information about the possible complications of surgery and radiotherapy choose aggressive management. Scientists involved in this field agree that the only way to determine the usefulness of early detection measures as a health care policy is by doing randomised treatment and/or randomised screening studies with cancer mortality as an endpoint. This rationale does not seem to determine medical practice at the moment. While this author very strongly feels that a randomised screening study comparing the 3 available tests to no screening should be conducted, it cannot be denied that in urological practice and by patients involved the possibility of overtreatment as outlined above is accepted to escape the risk of dying from cancer of the prostate.

REFERENCES

1   Catalona WJ, Smith DS, Ratliff TL, et al: Measurements of prostate-specific antigen in serum as a screening test for prostate cancer. N Engl J Med 1991 (324):1156-1161

2   Cooner WH, Mosley BR, Rutherford CJ Jr, Beard JH, Pond HS, Terry WJ, Igel TC, Kidd DD: Prostate cancer detection in a clinical urological practice by ultrasonography, digital rectal examination and prostate specific antigen. J Urol 1990 (143):1146-1154

3   Prorok PC, Connor RJ and Baker SG: Statistical considerations in cancer screening programs. Urol Clin North Am 1990 (17):699-708

4   Scardino PT, Weaver R and Hudson MA: Early detection of prostate cancer. Human Pathol 1992 (23):211-222

5   Schröder FH and Boyle P: Screening for prostate cancer - necessity or nonsense? Eur J Cancer 1993 (29A):656-661

6   Möller Jensen O, Esteve J, Möller H and Renard H: Cancer in the European community and its member states. Eur J Cancer 1990 (26):1167-1256

7   Breslow N, Chan CW, Dhom G, Drury RAB, Franks LM, Gellei B, Lee YS, Lundberg S, Sparke B, Sternby NH and Tulinius H: Latent carcinoma of prostate at autopsy in seven areas. Int J Cancer 1977 (20):680-688

8   Coebergh JWW: Incidence and prognosis of cancer in the Netherlands. Doctoral Thesis Erasmus University Rotterdam 1991

9   Lee F, Littrup PJ, Loft-Christensen L, Kelly BS, McHugh TA, Siders DB, Mitchell AE and Newby JE: Predicted prostate specific antigen results using transrectal ultrasound gland volume. Cancer (suppl.) 1992 (70):211-220

10 Schröder FH, Carpentier PJ, Maksimovic PA, et al: Transrectal ultrasonography (TRUS) - Volumetric applications to prostatic carcinoma. In: Resnick M, Watanabe H, Karr JP (eds) Diagnostic Ultrasound of the Prostate. Elsevier, New York 1989 pp 124-128

11 Carter HB, Morrell CH, Pearson JD, Brant LJ, Plato CC, Metter EJ, Chan DW, Fozard JL and Walsh PC: Estimation of prostatic growth using serial prostate-specific antigen measurements in men with and without prostate disease. Cancer Res 1992 (52[12]):3323-2238

12 Petros JA and Catalona WJ: Lower incidence of unsuspected lymph node metastases in 521 consecutive patients with clinically localized prostate cancer. J Urol 1992 (147):1574-1775

13 Franks LM: Latent carcinoma of the prostate. J Pathol Bacteriol 1954 (68):603-616

14 Mettlin C, Lee F, Drago J, Murphy GP: The American Cancer Society National Prostate Cancer Detection Project. Cancer 1991 (67):2949-2958

15 Schröder FH: The natural history of incidental prostatic carcinoma. In: Altwein JE, Faul P and Schneider W (eds) Incidental Carcinoma of the Prostate. Springer-Verlag, Berlin 1991 pp 56-62

16 Gaynor EP: Zur Frage des Prostatakrebs. Virchows Arch (A) 1938 (301):602-652

17 Bentvelsen FM and Schröder FH: Modalities available for screening for prostate cancer. Eur J Cancer 1993 (29A):804-811

18 Thompson IM and Zeidman EJ: Current urological practice: routine urological examination and early detection of carcinoma of the prostate. J Urol 1992 (148):326-329

Endocrine Aspects of Prostate Cancer

K. Griffiths[1], M.E. Harper[1], C.L. Eaton[1], A. Turkes[1] and W.B. Peeling[2]

1 Tenovus Cancer Research Centre, University of Wales College of Medicine, Heath Park, Cardiff, Wales CF4 4XX, United Kingdom
2 Department of Urology, St Woolos Hospital, Newport, Gwent, United Kingdom

Prostatic cancer in the year 2000 will be at the forefront of medical problems affecting the male population of the world. There is now a considerable amount of evidence to indicate that cancer of the prostate gland is, or is quickly becoming, the most commonly diagnosed cancer in men in the western world. The incidence rate appears to be consistently rising and, interestingly, the mortality rate for the black population of the United States of America is double that of the white people. It is becoming very evident that prostatic disease, both benign prostatic hyperplasia (BPH) as well as cancer, has become a serious health-care problem, particularly when considered in relation to the ever increasing proportion of the population in the more developed countries that is over the age of 65 years.

The time is most appropriate to re-evaluate our understanding of the natural history of prostatic cancer and the molecular processes that are concerned with the pathogenesis of this disease. A similar reassessment of the clinical management of patients with prostatic cancer must also be worthwhile, with renewed emphasis being placed on the need for more innovative treatment options, the potential of which will clearly be highlighted as our knowledge of the molecular events associated with the initiation and progression of the disease increases.

Hormonal Therapy for Advanced Prostatic Cancer: Some Comments

The word "hormone" was used in public for the first time in 1905 by Sir Ernest Starling in his Croonian Lectures to the Royal College of Physicians, but it was perhaps fitting that the suggestion that the testes, like the thyroid gland, might produce some chemical substance which maintained the male characteristics, was voiced earlier at a series of 3 Hunterian Lectures by Dr. J. Griffiths in the late nineteenth century. It is generally accepted that our understanding of the testicular control of the accessary sex glands began with the observations of John Hunter around 1786, although at that time he did not interpret his results in terms of endocrine factors, a credit that should be attributed to Berthold. Among these famous names associated with the early history of endocrinology ranks Charles Huggins, whose early work around 1940 established the scientific basis for the treatment of advanced prostatic cancer by androgen ablative procedures. Over the past 50 years, his work relating to the androgen dependence of prostatic cancer has dominated most disciplines associated with prostatic studies, irrespective of whether they were concerned experimentally with growth regulatory processes, or responsible for the clinical management of patients with the disease. Huggins indicated that the symptoms and general well-being of men with advanced cancer could be improved by orchidectomy, or by use of the, then new, orally active diethylstilboestrol (DES). At that time, there was probably a real sense of hope among urologists. The fact that these new treatment regimens were based upon scientific studies relating to the physiological control of prostatic activity was surely ground for optimism that further advances in the management of the disease would, in time, follow.

Through most of these past 5 decades, orchidectomy and DES have provided the mainstay of treatment, with orchidectomy the "gold standard" against which other forms of therapy could be assessed. However, although 70% of patients with advanced disease do experience symptomatic relief with primary endocrine therapy, relapse is generally inevitable within 1-2 years, and median survival time is then 6 months. Despite this, there has been a massive commitment throughout these years to the "fine tuning" of endocrine treatment in the search for the most effective, but least troublesome and safest procedure.

Subcapsular orchidectomy, DES-diphosphate (Honvan), the intramuscular injectable, long-acting polyoestradiol phosphate (Estradurin), Premarin, the mixture of conjugated equine oestrogens and ethinyloestradiol have all had their proponents. There was very reasonable logic behind the use of the progestational steroids such as hydroxyprogesterone caproate (Delalutin), chlormadinone acetate, medroxyprogesterone acetate (Provera) and cyproterone acetate (Androcur), the dual action of which inhibited luteinising hormone (LH) release from the pituitary and also elicited an inhibitory effect on the intracellular binding of 5α-dihydrotestosterone (DHT) to its receptor at the target cell. Jack Geller would describe this approach as an exercise in "complete androgen blockade".

The past decade has seen a major innovation. Following the isolation and characterisation of LH-releasing hormone (LH-RH) by Andrew Schally, the various LH-RH analogues such as depot-Zoladex were developed. Zoladex, administered once monthly, was seen to be equally efficacious as castration for the management of advanced prostatic cancer [1]. The synthesis and secretion of testosterone by the testis can now be controlled by medical means, by agents with few if any significant side effects; but do the adrenal androgens, dehydroepiandrosterone (DHA) sulphate, DHA and androstenedione, which are certainly a source

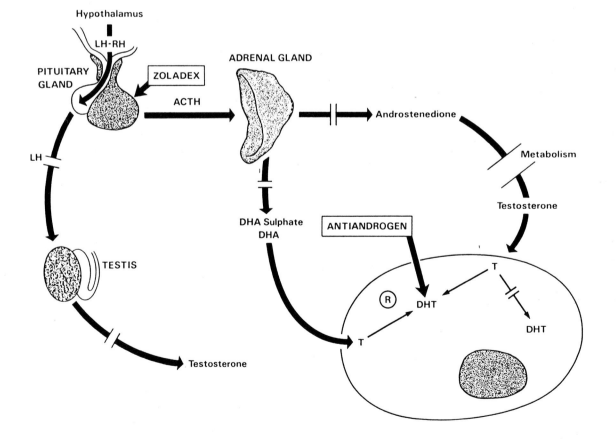

Fig. 1. Combination therapy - the "complete androgen blockade" - for the treatment of advanced prostatic cancer

of precursor steroid for the production of DHT within the prostate, play any role in promoting the continued growth and progression of prostatic cancer after primary endocrine therapy? Fernand Labrie evoked some early thoughts of Charles Huggins that both orchidectomy and adrenalectomy might be necessary to control advanced prostatic cancer. Professor Labrie introduced the "complete androgen blockade", an LH-RH analogue together with an antiandrogen as primary therapy, the antiandrogen regulating the molecular action of residual DHT at the target cell (Fig. 1). His early work provided a major stimulus to the field of urology, with a suggestion that the fine-tuning of the regimen for endocrine therapy was virtually complete and advanced prostatic cancer could be better controlled. The recent meeting in Paris, however, where the meta-analysis of data from more than 25 trials relating to such combination therapy was discussed, tended to indicate that with the patients introduced into these studies, combination treatment with LH-RH analogue and antiandrogen was no better than analogue alone. These studies are discussed later in this book by L. Denis.

Discussion at the meeting centred on whether sufficient patients had been included in the trials to produce the necessary data to highlight the differences between the groups. If the differences are so small to require such numbers, however, it might be argued that any benefits from combination therapy would be of little consequence.

Important issues still need to be considered. To many, the accumulated data would suggest that there probably is a subgroup of patients with more differentiated, less aggressive cancer, who could well benefit from complete androgen blockade. Possibly such patients could be much more critically selected for combination studies, using various clinical parameters and such currently available prognostic factors (Fig. 2) as Ki-67 and PCNA analysis [2] for recruitment into yet another, but more definitive trial, with emphasis placed on smaller numbers of carefully identified patients. Moreover, the degree of toxicity recorded for patients on antiandrogens suggests that the associated nausea and vomiting could mitigate against the accumulation of an effective intraprostatic concentration of the drugs. Some recent studies by De Jong and Schroeder in Rotterdam would certainly suggest that intranuclear prostatic levels of cyproterone acetate would not be particularly high. It would appear that better antiandrogens may well be required.

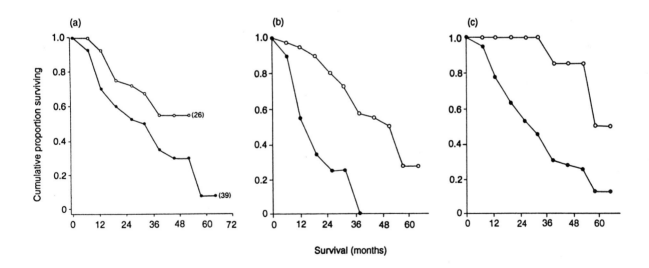

Fig. 2. PCNA and Ki-67 expression in prostatic cancer: relation to disease progression. (a) Relationship of PCNA scores of prostatic carcinoma and patient survival following diagnosis. Figures in parentheses indicate patient numbers: open circles relate to those patients whose PCNA score indicated less than 10% of nuclei stained, closed circles relate to patients whose score indicated more than 10% of nuclei positively stained. (b) Relationship of Ki-67 expression and survival, open circles relating to less than 1% of cells stained, n=52; closed circles, Ki-67 expression with more than 1% cells stained, n=31. Mantel-Cox and Breslow test p < 0.0001. (c) open circles, no Ki-67 expression, n=14; closed circles, Ki-67 expression positive in all tumours, n=69. Mantel-Cox and Breslow test p < 0.0001.

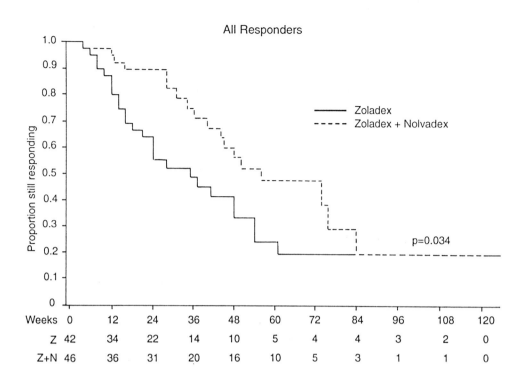

Fig. 3. Combination therapy for advanced cancer of the breast in pre- and perimenopausal women, life table analysis of duration of responce to endocrine therapy

Complete Oestrogen Blockade for Breast Cancer: Relevance to the Prostate

In this respect, it is of interest to consider the situation with regard to the management of carcinoma of the breast. Early studies of the Tenovus Institute in the late 1970s had established that Zoladex was equally effective as oophorectomy in regulating the growth of DMBA-induced mammary carcinoma in rats. Furthermore, joint studies of R. Nicholson of the Institute, with R. Blamey of the University of Nottingham Breast Clinic indicated not only that Zoladex was as effective as ovariectomy for the management of the pre- or perimenopausal women with advanced breast cancer, but that combination therapy with Zoladex, together with the antioestrogen tamoxifen, was more effective than Zoladex alone, not in terms of the proportion of patients that responded to therapy, but in time to disease progression (Fig. 3). Early results also indicate a possible benefit with regard to survival. More complete oestrogen blockade would appear of value for breast cancer therapy.

Tamoxifen, which acts as a partial agonist, has little, if any, toxicity and few side effects, and is invaluable for the treatment of advanced breast cancer in the postmenopausal woman. Of relevance, however, are current studies of R. Nicholson and D. Manning of the Tenovus Institute on the growth of oestrogen-responsive human breast MCF7 cancer cells in culture (Fig. 4). Addition of oestradiol stimulates growth - which is seen when the cancer cells are compared to the control cells - promoting proliferation as recognised by the Ki-67 antibody, which detects a nuclear protein expressed in cycling cells in G1, S, G2 and M phases, but not in the resting G0 phase. There is also an increased expression of oestrogen (ER) and progesterone (PgR) receptor proteins. Tamoxifen and 4-hydroxytamoxifen inhibit this stimulatory effect. Interesting, however, is the growth of the control cells in the apparent absence of oestrogen. Addition of ICI 164384, a pure antioestrogen without agonistic properties, inhibits the growth of the control cells. Moreover, studies on the effect of the antioestrogens on the expression of various recently cloned oestrogen-regulated genes, demonstrate the apparent complete switch-off of such

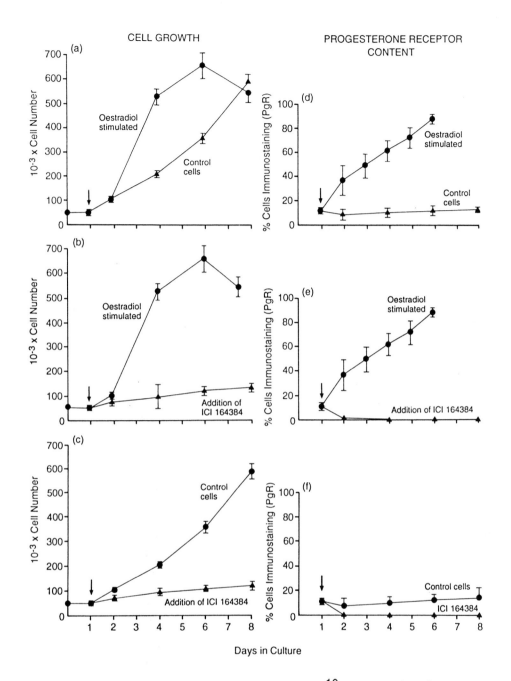

Fig. 4. MCF-7 breast cancer cells in culture: influence of oestradiol (10^{-10}M) on growth and on progesterone receptor (PgR) expression. Cells are grown in phenol red-free RPMI tissue culture medium containing charcoal-stripped foetal calf serum (5%). Tamoxifen addition restrained the rate of cell growth at the control level, whereas addition of ICI 164384 (10^{-7} M) inhibited growth and PgR expression.

genes by ICI 164384, and emphasise the partial oestrogenic effect of tamoxifen (Fig. 5).

Clearly, therefore, very low, undetectable levels of oestrogen, presumably in association with the appropriate growth regulatory factors, can support the growth of these hormone-responsive cells. Tamoxifen, although clinically a most valuable antioestrogen which very effec-

tively localises in breast tumour tissue in a 2000-fold excess over oestradiol levels, still fails to suppress oestrogen-regulated gene expression. The new pure antioestrogens, 7-alkylamide derivatives of oestradiol (Fig. 6), would appear most effective, certainly in culture, and clinical studies with such compounds are currently being established. The question

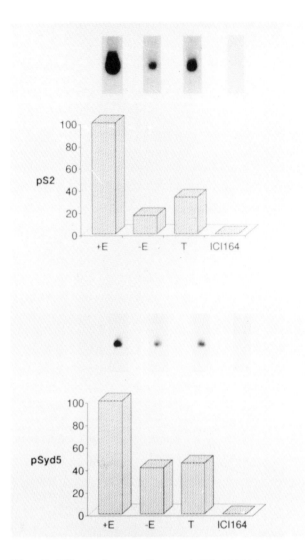

Fig. 5. Effect of tamoxifen and ICI 163384 on the expression of certain oestrogen-responsive genes. Northern blot analysis illustrates the partial agonistic effect of tamoxifen and the complete antagonistic action of ICI164384, the "pure" antioestrogen.

as to the potential of 7-alkylamide derivatives of DHT, or similar compounds, as pure antiandrogens should be raised, but it would certainly seem reasonable to consider that a search for less toxic, more effective antiandrogens would not be out of place.

Progression of Advanced Disease

The essential problem with the management of prostatic cancer is that the majority of patients present with a disease that has spread be-

yond the confines of the gland. The disease is then incurable with palliative endocrine therapy, the current first-line treatment. Disease progression expresses the inexorable, autonomous growth of clones of hormone-unresponsive cancer cells. This clonal selection after primary endocrine therapy results in tumour repopulation, and it seems very reasonable to believe that the rational approach to therapy must be to offer a combination hormonal-cytotoxic regimen immediately the cancer is diagnosed and when the number of androgen-independent cells is at a minimum.

An acceptable cytotoxic regimen has been difficult to identify however, and the associated clinical problems of such therapy are well recognised. A pragmatic approach is needed, possibly even the consideration of specific drug targeting using specific antibodies against prostatic cancer cells, with cytotoxic or radioactive agents attached. Some more recent work from the Tenovus Institute [3] tends to provide support for the potential of this concept. More specific targeting of cytotoxic agents linked to steroids could also be considered innovative and the development of Estracyt, a drug with a nor-nitrogen mustard attached as a carbamate to the C-3 atom of oestradiol, has provoked considerable interest. It does not appear to act as an alkylating agent and its precise place in the management of progressive disease still remains to be identified. Concurrent research in the Tenovus Institute in the late 1960s, possibly even preceding the announcement of Estracyt, related to the attachment of nitrogen mustard groups to DES and also to tamoxifen, a concept taken up by ICI Pharmaceuticals: the compounds were referred to as ICI 85966 and ICI 79792 (Fig. 6), respectively. Unfortunately, little time has been available to commit to their evaluation.

The need to recognise early prostatic cancer is now established and it has provided the necessary stimulus to the development of screening initiatives or better health-care programmes for men. If prostatic cancer is to be cured, the disease must be identified in its earlier stages of growth when confined to the gland. Such screening initiatives will also provide a complementary incentive to the establishment of appropriate investigations aimed to increase our understanding of the natural history of prostatic cancer and the molecular events associated with carcinogenic processes in the gland.

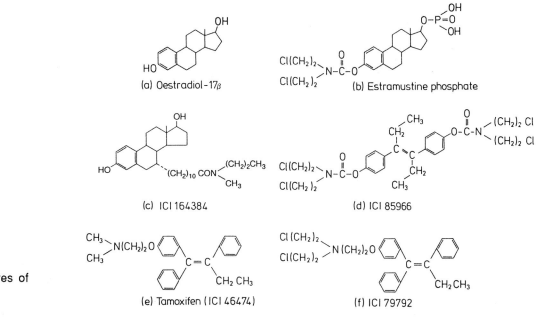

Fig. 6. Structures of various steroid antagonists

(a) Oestradiol-17β

(b) Estramustine phosphate

(c) ICI 164384

(d) ICI 85966

(e) Tamoxifen (ICI 46474)

(f) ICI 79792

Pathogenesis of Prostatic Cancer

Carcinogenesis is a complex, multi-step process from initiation, through promotion and progression to the invasive metastatic cancer (Fig. 7), with new information appearing regularly with regard to the molecular events relating to these changes. The search for early prostatic cancer can do nothing but good in the

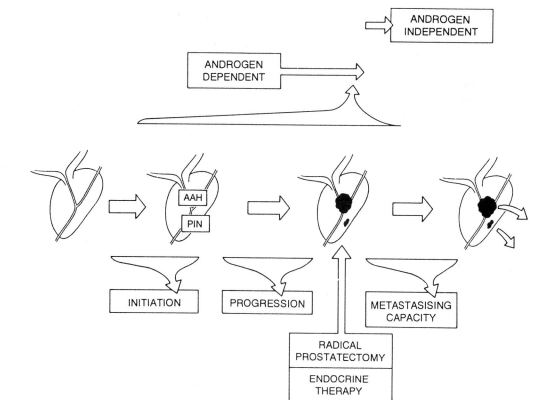

Fig. 7. Diagrammatic representation of prostate cancer development

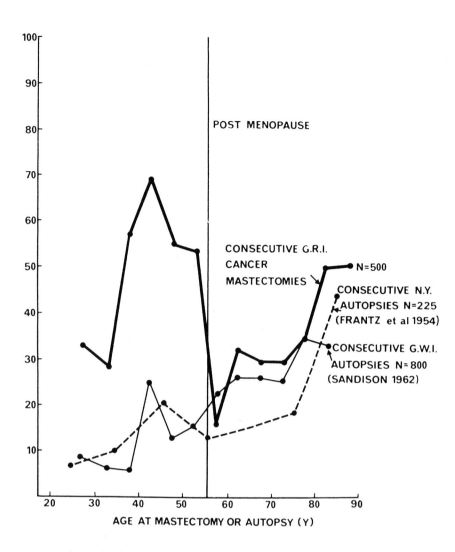

POST MENOPAUSE

CONSECUTIVE G.R.I.
CANCER
MASTECTOMIES

N=500

CONSECUTIVE N.Y.
AUTOPSIES N=225
(FRANTZ et al 1954)

CONSECUTIVE G.W.I.
AUTOPSIES N= 800
(SANDISON 1962)

AGE AT MASTECTOMY OR AUTOPSY (Y)

Fig. 8. The age-frequency distribution of hyperplasia in breast cancer mastectomies compared to autopsy controls. In the consecutive autopsies, there is an age-related increase in the prevalence of hyperplasia. In the consecutive cancer mastectomies, this prevalence is higher in the premenopausal age group. Data for the autopsy studies are from Glasgow Royal Infirmary, Sandison, A.T. NCI Monogr, US Dept. HEW, 1962 (81):1-145, and from Frantz et al., Cancer 1954 (4):762-783, 1954.

promotion of this research and the provision of appropriate material to investigate the pathogenesis of the disease. It is now accepted that approximately 75% of cancers originate in the peripheral zone of the gland, but that 25% develop in the centrally located transition zone, often identifiable in transurethral resection currettings removed at prostatectomy for BPH. The frequency with which cancer is found incidentally rises with increasing age. Furthermore, although incidental cancer was once considered an early phase in the natural history of prostatic cancer, a lesion of low intrinsic malignant potential, progressive disease is now reported for nearly a third of patients with stage T1b cancer, a frequency higher than that for stage T2a cancers palpated rectally. Moreover, after radical prostatectomy for T1b or T2a cancer, those patients with T1b disease were more likely to have a more aggressive cancer with metastatic spread to the lymph nodes. Despite these cancers being considered "latent", small

and well differentiated, eliciting little cause for concern, 16% of T1a cancers have been reported to progress, with time, to metastatic disease.

But what of premalignancy? John McNeal describes an age-related increase in atypical hyperplasia, a diffuse or multifocal proliferation of ductal or epithelial tissue, which he has related to premalignancy. These lesions are more prevalent in tissue with cancer than in controls and they would appear to have a close similarity to the increased incidence of epitheliosis and fibrocystic disease of breast epithelial tissue (Fig. 8), again more prevalent in premenopausal breasts with cancer than in controls [4]. Both premalignant conditions would appear to be influenced by age-related endocrine parameters.

The multifocal origin of prostate cancer is of interest, the propensity to develop predominantly in the peripheral zone requires consideration and the question now most effectively raised by Dr. David Bostwick as to whether BPH is causally related to a subgroup of cancers originating in the transition zone, must be addressed. There is a similarity in the natural history of BPH and cancer, both showing an increasing prevalence with aging, although that for BPH is evident a number of years earlier than that for cancer. BPH and cancer originate as hormone-dependent conditions which fail to develop in men castrated early in life, i.e., before puberty. Resected tissue at prostatectomy for BPH contains atypical adenomatous hyperplasia (AAH), which, like prostatic intraepithelial neoplasia (PIN), accepted as a premalignant lesion in the peripheral zone, possibly should also be similarly considered an early phase in the escape of epithelial proliferation from growth regulatory processes. AAH presents as foci of small glands reminiscent of well differentiated adenocarcinoma.

Some Aspects of the Molecular Endocrinology of the Normal Prostate

With regard to the aetiology of prostatic disease, both BPH and cancer, two parameters have consistently been recognised as exercising some degree of influence over disease processes: 1) the presence of the testes and 2) an aging factor. As emphasised earlier, neither BPH nor cancer develop in men castrated prior to puberty, DHT would certainly appear to be a necessary and important factor in the pathogenesis of BPH, and the prevalence of both diseases increases after the age of 50.

The molecular processes by which androgens influence prostatic growth are less well understood than those concerned with the regulation of the secretory protein genes. Androgens are essential since the prostate cannot develop, differentiate, nor maintain size or function in their absence. The adult prostate does not grow in response to exogenous androgen administration but maintains its normal size through a balance between agonistic effects on the proliferative processes of cell renewal and an antagonistic effect of androgen on cell death. Depletion of androgen receptor (AR) instigates involution, reaccumulation of AR initiates proliferation, and administration of testosterone to immature male rats accelerates prostatic growth, but only until the gland attains normal maximal size. The synthesis of nuclear AR is in synchrony neither with the initiation nor with the shut-down of DNA synthesis and it would appear that androgens are essential, but not primarily responsible for prostatic cell proliferation. Androgens "switch on" growth processes, but the intercession of the various intermediary growth regulatory factors would seem necessary.

Overlaid on this steady state of homeostasis, with the rate of cell proliferation balanced by an equal rate of cell death, is the interactive relationship that exists between the stromal and epithelial elements of the prostate, so elegantly demonstrated by the studies of Gerry Cunha. It would appear that androgen-dependent mediators of stromal origin regulate growth processes in the epithelium (Fig. 9). The observed mitogenic effects of androgens on prostatic explants containing both epithelial and stromal tissue, a response not seen with isolated epithelial cells in culture, would be explained by the androgen-dependent role of the stroma in producing growth regulating factors that influence the epithelium. Dr Sammy Franks tried to explain this phenomenon to us, many years ago!

It would generally be accepted that the growth of the prostate from a pea-sized gland at the age of 10, to the walnut size of the mature, adult, 20 g organ at 20-25 years of age, essentially involves the laying down of 40-50 epithelial-lined ducts in a bed of stromal tissue. This epithelial growth ceases in the early 20s, and it must be presumed that a molecular shut-down mechanism overrides these growth promoting effects when homeostasis is established. Expressed simply, this could involve a balance between the growth promoting effects of epidermal growth factor (EGF), fibroblast growth factor (FGF) and insulin-like growth factor (IGF), for example, and the growth restraining influence of transforming growth factor (TGF)ß, the latter preventing overgrowth. Microscopic BPH, recognised in the late 20s, and increasing in prevalence with increasing age in men of all races from both the eastern and western regions of the world, could well be perceived as the consequence of an imbalance, whereby the proliferative factors override the growth inhibitory influences.

Other factors must, however, be considered with regard to the regulation of prostatic growth;

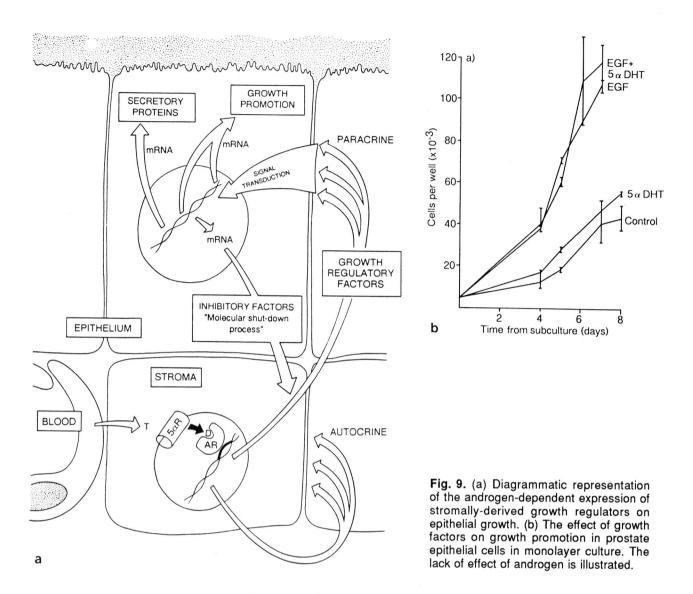

Fig. 9. (a) Diagrammatic representation of the androgen-dependent expression of stromally-derived growth regulators on epithelial growth. (b) The effect of growth factors on growth promotion in prostate epithelial cells in monolayer culture. The lack of effect of androgen is illustrated.

the recent, innovative studies of Chung Lee in Chicago highlight certain aspects of the complexity of these multi-hormonal regulatory processes. Relative to the distance from the urethra, he describes regions of the glandular ductal system as proximal, intermediate and distal segments. Professor Lee identified a distinct regional variation in both the morphology and functional activity of the epithelial cells. The distal complements were actively proliferating, those in the intermediate region were differentiated and secreting protein, whereas those in the proximal segment were associated with programmed cell death, the latter exclusively expressing sulphated glycoprotein-2 (SGP-2), an androgen-suppressed gene product identical to the castration-induced protein, testosterone-repressed prostatic message-2, and to the

protein that has been termed clusterin. The differential expression of this androgen-repressed gene product among the epithelial cells of the ductal system paradoxically occurs in the presence of normal circulating levels of androgens, indicating a regional variation in the response of the epithelial cells to androgens, or to androgen-dependent growth regulatory factors, some possibly of stromal origin.

Chung Lee's studies provide a fascinating new dimension to normal growth regulation in the prostate and could provide the basis for understanding the loss of control in what would seem to be the locally-biased process concerned with the random focal development of microscopic epithelial hyperplasia and micro-epithelial nodules in the transition zone of the prostate, the signs of early BPH.

Growth Regulatory Systems: Potential for Imbalance

Information on the complex inductive, inter- and intracellular signalling processes in the prostate is rapidly accumulating [5] and concepts as to how they regulate growth are being established; their relationship to abnormal growth, both benign and cancer, can be envisaged. Impairment of these multi-component systems could readily provoke abnormal growth, with the intrinsic fine-regulation overridden by an imbalance of factors, some of which may be related to aging.

Prostate-derived growth factors have been identified in normal and abnormal prostatic tissues and secretions. It is now accepted that EGF and TGFα have mitogenic effects on isolated prostatic epithelial cells in culture, growth promotion being exercised through EGF receptors (EGF-R) located in the cell membrane. Another growth promoting factor with a high affinity for heparin, and identified as a member of the endothelial cell growth factor family, is basic FGF. It remains to be established whether bFGF is implicated only in stromal growth, or whether it also influences prostatic epithelial cells.

Human prostate-derived fibroblasts produce bFGF which stimulates their own growth in an autocrine manner. Moreover, fibroblasts stimulate the clonal growth of human prostate epithelial cells and FGF is reported to have mitogenic effects on epithelial cells in culture. Interestingly, it would appear that FGF production by fibroblasts is regulated by TGFß, not by androgens. Also noteworthy are studies in which T. Thompson introduced, in a transgenic model system and regulated by a viral promoter, the int-2 proto-oncogene, a member of the FGF family. The high level expression of this gene in the prostates of male mice was accompanied by significant epithelial hyperplasia of the prostate.

High-affinity receptors for insulin and the IGFs, or somatomedins, are also present in the prostate and IGF-1 is also mitogenic. The restraining influence of TGFß on epithelial cell proliferation is also well recognised, with evidence available to indicate that TGFß mRNA and TGFß-receptor expression are repressed by androgen, but elevated during castration-induced, programmed cell death. Do androgens influence FGF production through their regulatory effect on TGFß expression? The synthesis of EGF by the rat ventral prostate is reported to require androgens, whereas its secretion is modulated by α-adrenergic control. Furthermore, EGF-R expression is normally down-regulated by androgens, again suggesting a finely regulated control mechanism.

These growth regulatory mechanisms are clearly modulated by androgens, but there also appears to be a role for oestrogens, the action of which seems stromally biased and could be implicated, synergistically with androgens, in the pathogenesis of clinically symptomatic BPH, which manifests extensive stromal hyperplasia.

Initiation of Prostatic Cancer

Effective communication between cells by means of chemical information, the accurate deciphering of the information and the precise response elicited to it, are all part and parcel of the complex growth regulatory processes. The realisation that the oncogenes of the acutely transforming retroviruses are transduced cognates of normal genes [6], cellular proto-oncogenes which are normally concerned in growth regulation and differentiation, has now allowed a greater insight into the consequences of their impairment. Oncogenes, therefore, are normal growth regulatory genes in which alterations of structure or expression have occurred, and it is now recognised that all cellular genes encoding components of systems that are concerned with growth or differentiation, must be considered as proto-oncogenes. Furthermore, amplification, mutation or translocation of such genes could lead to malignant transformation of the cells harbouring the altered genes [6].

The search for aberrant genes in prostatic cancer would appear daunting, yet it is very reasonable to believe that a judicious screening of tumour samples could direct attention to anomalous gene expression, alterations that may be implicated in the initiation of cancer and in the escape from hormone regulation.

The concept of multi-step carcinogenesis relates to a succession of stages in which particular proto-oncogenes are activated, each step inducing changes consistent with the development of the appropriate phenotype necessary for transformation, thereby conferring full malignant potential. R. Weinberg [7] introduced a "two-oncogene" concept whereby two complementary oncogenes, for example *ras*, encoding cytoplasmic proteins and *myc*, encoding nuclear proteins, could, when transfected together, elicit a full cancer phenotype. Although transformation can be induced by transfection of a single oncogene into NIH3T3 cells, for example, thereby inducing growth factor expression and anchorage independence, it was realised that the characteristics of immortalisation, conferred by *myc* transfection, are already intrinsic, established parameters of such cells, which might be considered a "premalignant phenotype". Also relevant are studies in which somatic cell hybridisation demonstrates the presence of growth inhibiting genes, the fusion of normal with tumour cells producing, in the hybrid cells, a restricted tumourigenicity. Such tumour suppressor genes are concerned in the regulation of normal growth, and their loss removes their inhibitory effect on cell proliferation.

Simply, therefore, carcinogenesis concerns the complementary "misbehaviour" of various oncogenes and tumour suppressor genes, oncogene activation resulting from mutation, amplification or re-arrangement, and deletion or mutation leading to the loss of suppressor gene expression. Genetic changes relating to the activation of cellular proto-oncogenes must be sought. This, together with the recognition of growth regulatory factors that are facultatively expressed under androgen influence, but constitutively expressed when autonomy is achieved, will provide a greater insight into the factors sustaining the promotion and progression of prostatic cancer.

Cytogenetic analysis of prostatic cancer by Dr Peehl and her colleagues identified certain chromosome deletions and structural changes. Although there were few patients in the study, they directed attention to deletions associated with chromosomes 10q and 7q. Dr Carter and his colleagues in Johns Hopkins, Baltimore, using allelotyping and polymorphic DNA probes, provided good evidence for the specificity of allelic deletions on chromosomes 10 and 16 of prostatic cancer. Such technology identified in colorectal tumours the frequent deletion of the long arm of chromosome 17,

thereby allowing the recognition of p53 as a tumour suppressor gene, inactivated in this particular cancer. Evidence directs attention to the central role that p53 may have in various forms of human cancer, and later studies of Dr Carter indicated that 25% of prostatic cancers examined showed evidence of allelic deletion on chromosome 17p and 13q, the locations of p53 and retinoblastoma (Rb) genes, respectively.

A mutant protein, expressed as a result of an exon deletion of the Rb gene, has been identified in the DU145 prostatic cancer cell line. Moreover, transfection of the cloned normal Rb gene into DU145 cells in nude mice suppressed tumourigenicity. The aberrant Rb protein has not yet been detected in other prostatic cancer cell lines, although the analysis of human prostatic cancer samples indicated a deletion of 103 nucleotides from the Rb gene promoter region of one tumour.

The Early Phases of Prostatic Carcinogenesis

It is clearly important to pinpoint anomalies in the expression of genes known to be fundamental to the complex cascade of molecular events that are mobilised by the growth factors and that influence the biology of prostatic growth. Gene alterations that could be implicated in the initiation of cancer of the prostate and in the escape from hormone dependence, can be identified in many of the pathways by which androgens both regulate growth and repress programmed cell death. Doubtless, many other genetic lesions could also contribute to carcinogenesis. It is important that we can identify precancerous lesions and their biological characteristics, thus providing the basis for the recognition of more effective targets for intervention therapy.

Deregulation of growth processes leading to hyperplasia would certainly seem to be implicated in early phases of premalignancy and the possible effects of an external carcinogen on this situation must always be recognised. It remains to be seen, however, whether the usurpation of its own growth regulatory mechanism confers on a cell a distinct advantage of operating in an autocrine mode. Can oncogene activation be identified in the foci of atypical hyperplasia described by John McNeal, or in AAH or PIN, premalignant lesions highlighted by David Bostwick? Abnormal clonal growth will proceed as a "premalignant phenotype", associated with an activated oncogene, but the restraining influence of the neighbouring normal cells will exercise an inhibitory effect over the growth of the aberrant cells. R. Weinberg [7] describes most succinctly the experimental approaches relating to the means by which small clones of premalignant cells expand despite the restraining influence of normal, neighbouring cells, thereby "transcending a hostile environment". He indicates that an activated *ras* oncogene is often observed in such early clones, suggesting that it could be one of the early factors in tumour formation.

Dr Trapman and his colleagues in Rotterdam have reported a consistently high expression of c-Ha-*ras* in a series of prostatic cancer cell lines. Studies from the Tenovus Cancer Research Centre indicated increasing levels of c-Ha-*ras* mRNA transcripts with tumour dedifferentiation, although Dr Varma has challenged the concept that high levels of the *ras* p21 protein can be used as a marker of tumour proliferation in prostatic cancer. Furthermore, despite John Isaacs demonstrating that transfection of an activated *ras* oncogene increases the metastatic potential of prostatic cancer cells, Dr Peehl would probably argue that activation of a *ras* oncogene *in situ* is a rare event in prostatic cancer. However, in an experimental system referred to as a mouse prostate reconstitution model, T. Thompson demonstrated that the introduction of *ras* and *myc* together induced an actively proliferating carcinoma of the prostate gland.

Escape from an inhibiting environmental influence can be experimentally forced by use of tumour promoters such as phorbol acetates [7], which are reported to reduce the gap junction-mediated communication between cells, thereby restraining the paracrine flow of growth inhibitory factors or signals from the normal to the "cancer-initiated" neighbour. At the same time, these tumour promoters stimulate protein kinase C (PK-C), an important component of the signal transduction processes transferring messages from membrane localised receptors for growth regulatory factors to the cell nucleus. Whereas studies from the Tenovus laboratories demonstrated an elevated level of c-*myc*

mRNA in prostatic cancer tissues of all grades of differentiation, those of Dr Buttyan reported increased c-*myc* expression only in less differentiated cancers. Nevertheless, detailed studies, centred on the activities of the c-*myc* and c-*fos* proto-oncogenes, would seem very reasonable, c-*fos* expression shown by ourselves to be closely correlated to AR levels in human prostatic cancer samples. The *fos* proto-oncogene appears to exercise a central role in growth regulation, turning on other genes in response to a wide range of stimuli. For example, the gene is activated by EGF and the phorbol esters, and its up-regulation is seen as one of the earliest nuclear responses, switching cells from G0 into cell cycle.

With studies [7] indicating that c-*myc* activation is necessary to allow *ras*-transformed embryo fibroblasts to override the inhibitory restraints of neighbouring cells, interest is directed to the normal control of the c-*myc* proto-oncogene. Expression of the normally quiescent c-*myc* gene is elevated in response to the stimulus of mitogenic signals elicited by growth promoting factors such as EGF. The cells then enter the cell cycle. It is very reasonable to envisage that the inhibitory influence of TGFß on epithelial cell proliferation is exercised through the suppression of the c-*myc* proto-oncogene, with TGFß expression modulated, to some degree at least, through its repression by androgens. Loss of the trans-acting growth inhibitory factors that normally shut down nuclear c-*myc*, or *myc*-like proto-oncogenes, or deletion of a *cis*-acting regulator, could allow constitutive expression of the proto-oncogene, or "oncogene status" [7]. Tumour suppressor genes, such as p53 and Rb, regulate normal proliferative processes by expression of their growth inhibitory proteins, and their deletion would remove this growth restraining effect. Introduction of the Rb gene into retinoblastoma cells restores normal growth control.

A direct induction of a proto-oncogene by androgens has yet to be demonstrated in the prostate, but Dr Weisz has shown that in the uterus oestrogens induce the expression of c-*fos*, c-*jun* and c-*myc*, and an oestrogen response element has been located upstream of the human c-*fos* gene, associated with core sequences for AP-1 transcription binding sites. The rapid response of the c-*fos* gene in the androgen-promoted regenerating prostate of the castrated rat, reported by Dr Buttyan, provides evidence that further studies with this proto-oncogene could be of value in relation to understanding the development of androgen independence.

Cancer Progression: Prognostic Factors, Metastatic Propensity

In a recent report from the 1991 International Consensus on BPH held in Paris, David Bostwick discussed the relationship of BPH to cancer, the urgent need to stage localised cancer and the prognostic importance of tumour volume, considered by some to be the most important prognostic factor in early prostatic cancer. Available data indicates that tumour volume and grade are strong predictors of progression. Although with frequent exceptions, tumours generally become less differentiated as they increase in size. The larger the tumour, the greater the incidence of capsular penetration and seminal vesicle invasion; capsular penetration is seen to be more prevalent with tumours between 0.5-1.0 cc, seminal vesicle invasion with 3 cc, and metastatic spread relating to a volume of 5 cc. Possibly important to bear in mind is the classical belief that a cancer cell after 27 doublings would reach a size of 2 mm (0.2 cc). Three subsequent doublings, and the cancer attains a size of 1 cc, or 1 gm; a further 10 produces a 1 kg tumour (1000 cc). It is interesting to consider the molecular events that relate to these phenomena and their potential as predictors of tumour development (Table 1), i.e., imbalance of the growth regulatory mechanisms leading to hyperplasia, genetic instability with gene activation, mutation or deletion, re-

lates to cancer initiation. This may be followed by steady growth and progression. Some prostatic cancers would appear to remain latent, however, with a prevalence at the age of 50, in the prostates of men of all races, from East and West, of the order of 30%. Current information relating to the presentation of prostatic cancer in the western countries would suggest that approximately 1% of these latent cancers progress, to eventually present clinically as advanced disseminated disease. Approximately 10% of prostatic cancers are, however, recognised at prostatectomy for BPH.

In relation to size, J. Folkman [8] indicates that new capillary blood vessels are necessary for a tumour to expand beyond 2 mm, so that angiogenesis must then play an important role in determining further growth and dissemination. Assessment of the microvessels at the margins of breast carcinoma have recently been reported to be valuable predictors of metastasis. P. Gullino, in the late 1970s, suggested that angiogenesis could be a preneoplastic marker, involved in the early phases of transformation to the malignant phenotype. Angiogenesis involves the growth towards the cancer of capillary sprouts, columns of endothelial cells from pre-existing capillaries, a process promoted by tumour expression of growth factors, probably FGF, the most potent angiogenic factor presently known. Under normal conditions such capillary growth would be regulated by a balance between endothelial cell growth factors, like FGF, and restraining factors such as TGFß. The blocking of angiogenesis would offer a potential therapeutic approach to inhibit tumour progression, and of interest are Folkman's reports that a decrease in size and metastatic capacity of tumours in experimental animals

Table 1. Tumour diagnosis and patient survival. Effect of doubling time

Tumour doubling time	Time to reach diagnosis size (1 g) (30 doublings)		Time to death (1000 g/1 kg) (40 doublings)		Life survival from diagnosis (30-40 doublings)	
Days	Days	Years	Days	Years	Days	Years
20	600	1.6	800	2.2	200	0.6
60	1800	4.9	2400	6.6	600	1.7
180	5400	14.7	7200	19.7	1800	5.0
240	7200	19.7	9600	26.3	2400	6.6

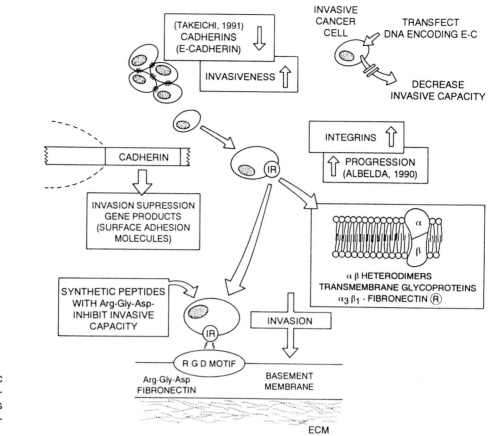

Fig. 10. Diagrammatic representation of the relationship of cadherins and integrins to the processes of metastasis

follows the administration of high-dose cortisone and heparin. There is also some indication that certain lesser known steroids like 11-epicortisol may be implicated in these processes as "angiostatic steroids". It would be interesting to know if an up-regulation of FGF expression could be recognised in those microfoci of premalignancy or early prostatic cancer. Other factors must be involved. Malignant cells have a reduced ability to adhere to each other, facilitating detachment and increased invasive potential. The cadherins, cell surface glycoproteins and mediators of calcium-dependent, epithelial cell adhesion, would therefore seem worthy of study in relation to early prostatic cancer (Fig. 10). Studies by Dr Cyr and his colleagues in Quebec indicate that in the epididymis, E-cadherin expression is regulated by androgens. Down-regulation in the expression of the E-cadherin gene, or its deletion, may indicate early invasive propensity. Loss of E-cadherin expression in tumour cell lines relates to the ability to invade collagen gels. Cadherins act therefore as invasion suppression gene products; furthermore, the gene is located

on chromosome 16q 22.1, chromosome 16 already being recognised as a site for allelic deletions in prostatic cancer.

The integrins require further study in relation to the prostate. The interaction between the migrating, invasive malignant cell and the adhesive proteins of the extracellular matrix (ECM) are mediated through integrins. Essentially, they are recognised as receptor proteins, transmembrane glycoprotein heterodimers, α and ß-subunits, the particular composition of which determines the component of the basement membrane of the ECM to which the cell can become re-attached. The $\alpha3,\beta1$-protein recognises a specific amino-acid sequence, an -Arg-Gly-Asp- motif, within the fibronectin molecule of the basement membrane. Synthetic peptides with this sequence of amino acids have been considered a possible approach to therapy, by inhibiting this attachment process. The integrin-mediated attachment of the malignant cell to the recognition motif of fibronectin therefore becomes an early step before the breakdown of the ECM allows cancer invasion to proceed. Up-regulation of the integrins has been related in some cancers to tumour aggressiveness and disease progression, although this is not an inevitable association. Further studies in relation to the prostate would seem reasonable.

Some exciting and innovative studies of L. Liotta [9] have been directed to the metastatic characteristics of malignant cells and the processes of capsule penetration, cancer dissemination and invasion. For the basement membrane to be degraded, proteolysis of these tissue barriers becomes an essential feature of invasion, with the cancer cells producing enzymes which degrade collagen. These collagenases are referred to as metalloproteinases. However, the cancer cells secrete not only the metalloproteinases, but also "tissue inhibitors of metalloproteinases", TIMP-1 and TIMP-2, that bind to and inhibit the collagenases. TIMPs would be considered "metastasis suppression gene products". The capacity of the cancer to express metalloproteinases and TIMPs would reflect metastatic propensity, deregulation of the balance in favour of the metalloproteinases promoting invasion. Professor Liotta, in highlighting the complexity of metastasis, also describes the expression of a gene nm23 in non-metastasising experimental mouse melanoma cells. In corresponding metastatic cells the gene is missing and the nm23 protein is deficient or absent. Again, the nm23 gene product acts as a suppressor of metastasis. Investigations with human breast cancer indicate high levels of nm23 in non-invasive cancers and low concentrations associated with metastatic spread and poor survival. Of the breast cancers studied, 50% were missing one of the two copies of the nm23 gene. The expression of the nm23 gene therefore correlates strongly with the propensity of the cancer to invade and disseminate, and again, studies of this gene in prostatic cancer would not seem irrelevant.

Important in these complex processes are the motility factors. Although certain growth regulators also influence cell motility, the motogenic cytokines would seem to be concerned primarily with cell movement. In normal physiology, cells migrate, for example, in relation to wound healing or inflammation, but the process is controlled. Deregulation would appear to be associated with cancer and tumour invasion. Scatter factor (SF), autocrine motility factor (AMF) and migration stimulating factor (MSF) have been reported to influence the motility of various epithelial cells. SF is secreted by fibroblasts and has a direct paracrine effect on cell movement. The secretion of SF by tumours has yet to be reported, although Professor Liotta describes the production of AMF by human melanoma cells such that it enhanced the cells' own mobility. There is evidence that the development of the aggressive, invasive cancer phenotype is accompanied by enhanced AMF expression relating to pseudopodia formation by the cell prior to migration. G-proteins and adenylate cyclase may be concerned in the transduction of the AMF signal received at the membrane-located AMF receptor: a consequent response would be the up-regulation of the integrins, receptors for fibronectin and laminin, the cell-substrate adhesion molecules. Also noteworthy is the report that cells of the mouse NIH3T3 embryonic cell line do not release AMF until transfected with *ras*-oncogene. Cell traction has been simply portrayed (Fig. 11) as a cell-substrate adhesion in the foremost, leading region of the migrating cell, and cell-substrate de-adhesion in the trailing aspect. MSF is produced by foetal, but not adult fibroblasts, although tumour-derived fibroblasts act like foetal cells. It is reported that skin fibroblasts from women with familial breast cancer express MSF, as do fibroblasts from a large proportion of first-degree relatives.

Prostatic Cancer: Progression to Androgen Resistance

The role of oncogenes is directed primarily towards cancer initiation, with their positive growth stimulating effects overriding normal growth regulatory signals generated by the androgens. The current research commitment to the study of cellular oncogenes will undoubtedly provide a greater understanding of prostatic carcinogenesis and, moreover, a better insight into potential prognostic indicators. Screening initiatives will identify "early cancer" and it is imperative that potential tumour behaviour can be recognised at this stage so that appropriate clinical management can be invoked. Any early influence of androgens over the facultative expression of the various growth factors may be lost as autonomy is re-

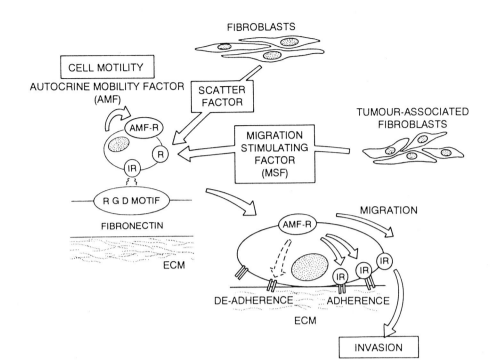

Fig. 11. Diagrammatic representation of the influence of motogenic factors on prostate cancer cell invasion

alised and growth factors are then constitutively expressed. A feature of prostatic cancer progression is the change from an androgen-dependent to an apparently faster growing, androgen-resistant phenotype, inferring some particular growth advantage to the latter.

It is perhaps appropriate, therefore, that in finalising this simple overview, some attention is directed to the concept of androgen sensitivity. It is generally stated that androgen-dependent cells die in the absence of hormone; androgen-sensitive cells survive, however, but grow more quickly in their presence. Some cells may be indirectly dependent on androgens, requiring paracrine growth promoting factors from neighbouring androgen-sensitive cells. Others may be insensitive to androgens. Extensive experience of breast cancer cells in culture would provoke Dr Roger King to emphasise that cultured breast cancer cells, deprived of steroid, invoke changes associated with the assumption of an oestrogen-unresponsive status, the changes generating genetic variants which proliferate more rapidly. Such changes are, in the short term, reversible, but after a longer period the cells cannot be stimulated by steroids.

Aneuploidy, genetic instability in a subpopulation of cells of a growing cancer could readily lead to the formation of cell variants with different degrees of androgen sensitivity. A complete deletion of the AR gene could be involved, this being recognised as one cause of androgen insensitivity syndrome, an X-chromosome-linked disorder characterised by defective masculinisation in karyotypically 46XY subjects with intra-abdominal or inguinal testes. A single basepair mutation and the deletion of the exons encoding the steroid binding domain of the AR have also been reported in association with the syndrome and it is clear that AR mutants may well be implicated in the changes relating to the loss of androgen sensitivity of prostatic cancer. At the same time, other biochemical or molecular events could be suggested. Hypermethylation of androgen response elements sited upstream of androgen-regulated genes could deregulate AR control of gene transcription. Furthermore, it must also be recognised that a mutant AR may not be androgen regulated, but could influence growth regulatory processes by its uncontrolled constitutive activation of androgen-responsive genes, an effect that could be promoted by various other growth regulators. P. Chambon [10] has described such events and the molecular biology which supports the concept.

It is reasonable to presume that prostatic cancer, diagnosed and recognised by the urologist, is a heterogeneous population of cell variants.

A large proportion of men who present with disseminated disease respond well to androgen-ablative therapy, a treatment, therefore, that will affect the growth of androgen-dependent and androgen-sensitive cells. Would there be a more effective response, with an extended time to relapse, if an effective complete androgen blockade could be instigated? The approach, which may be optimistic, may well require some new forms of antiandrogen therapy, thereby restraining the process of adaptation of a primarily androgen-sensitive cancer? Possibly even more pragmatic: what is the potential of conservative treatment of suitably identified, confined early prostatic cancer, with the new 5α-reductase inhibitors such as finasteride (Merck & Co. Inc.) and epristeride (Smith, Kline & Beecham)? Would a 5α-reductase, together with low-dose antiandrogen, offer complete androgen blockade?

A secondary issue revolves around the effect of such inhibitors on the progression of latent cancer, or early premalignant changes, in the prostates of men with early symptoms of bladder outflow obstruction who are receiving 5α-reductase inhibitors as intervention therapy.

The possibility of achieving complete DHT blockade by use of a 5α-reductase inhibitor in association with a less toxic, low dose of one of the currently available antiandrogens to inhibit the androgenic action of the residual intraprostatic DHT concentration could well offer another reasonable approach for the next decade, but whatever happens, we move into an exciting period that is providing a whole new molecular dimension to our understanding of the endocrine and biochemical processes that regulate prostatic growth and function. We can do nothing but once again feel a new sense of optimism pervading the laboratories and clinics of the "prostate people".

REFERENCES

1 Turkes AO, Peeling WB and Griffiths K: Treatment of patients with advanced cancer of the prostate: Phase III trial, Zoladex against castration; a study of the British Prostate Group. J Steroid Biochem 1987 (27):543-549

2 Harper ME, Glynne-Jones E, Goddard L, Wilson DW, Matenhelia SS, Conn IG, Peeling WB and Griffiths K: Relationship of proliferating cell nuclear antigen (PCNA) in prostatic carcinomas to various clinical parameters. The Prostate 1992 (20):243-253

3 Rowland AJ, Harper ME, Wilson DW and Griffiths K: The effect of an anti-membrane antibody-methotrxate conjugate on the human prostatic tumour line PC3. Br J Cancer 1990 (61):702-708

4 Simpson HW, Mutch F, Halberg F, Griffiths K and Wilson DW: Bimodal age-frequency distribution of epitheliosis in cancer mastectomies. Relevance to preneoplasia. Cancer 1982 (50):2417-2422

5 Griffiths K, Davies P, Eaton CL, Harper ME, Turkes A and Peeling WB: Endocrine factors in the initiation, diagnosis and treatment of prostatic cancer. In: Voigt KD and Knabbe C (eds) Endocrine Dependent Tumors. Raven Press Ltd, New York 1991 pp 83-130

6 Bishop JM: Cellular oncogenes and retroviruses. Ann Rev Biochem 1983 (52):301-354

7 Weinberg RA: Oncogenes, antioncogenes, and the molecular bases of multistep carcinogenesis. Cancer Res 1989 (49):3713-3721

8 Folkman, J: Toward an understanding of angiogenesis: search and discovery. Perspect in Biol and Med 1985 (29):10-36

9 Liotta LA, Steeg PS and Stetler-Stevenson WG: Cancer metastasis and angiogenesis: an imbalance of positive and negative regulation. Cell 1991 (64):327-336

10 Green S and Chambon P: Nuclear receptors enhance our understanding of transcription regulation. Trends Genet 1988 (4):309-314

The Diagnosis and Staging of Prostate Cancer

Gerald P. Murphy

American Cancer Society, 1599 Clifton Road N.E., Atlanta, Georgia 30329, U.S.A.

The grading and staging of prostate cancer has been an international obsession for urologists and pathologists for some time. After considerable and appropriate discussion in 1992, the TNM staging system for prostate cancer appears currently to be settled to the satisfaction of most (Table 1). As will be reported and described later in this review, however, the utilisation of the TNM system remains poor in some areas, especially in the United States.

Staging and grading has been part of the evaluation of response to treatment that various cooperative groups have employed to report results. The National Prostatic Cancer Project (NPCP) in 1972 had to institute further such therapeutic results. These criteria, as they existed in 1985, are summarised in Tables 2, 3, 4 and 5.

Prostate-specific antigen (PSA) from 1981 onwards was also measured in these studies and separately reported [2]. While the NPCP results have been disappointing, few have found fault with the stringent criteria of response employed. There are differences in the use of the stable category; however, the manner of the NPCP reporting has permitted all to address this issue based on evaluation of the NPCP results. For advanced disease today and in the future, markers such as PSA or others we have discovered can easily be substituted for acid phosphatase and/or alkaline phosphatase [3,4].

Early disease, in contrast to more advanced, is a difficult evaluation problem. In studies where chemotherapy agents are being administered as adjuvants to surgery or radiotherapy - that is meant to be definitive in that all signs of disease are clinically removed or eradicated - the measure of response is based on recurring disease. This can be tabulated as recurrence rates at given time intervals or presented as reverse life table curves of recurrences or as distributions of disease-free intervals. Survival analysis is usually performed, but the post-recurrence treatment effects can confound treatment comparisons. These and other factors can affect the outcome of adjuvant studies and some examples are presented in Table 6. For these reasons such studies take longer time to complete, require more patients, and are more difficult to evaluate.

Evidence of recurrence in early disease following definitive procedures for prostate cancer obviously presents differences of opinion, particularly regarding the clinical necessity for biopsies in critical areas, e.g. lungs and liver. In general, however, biopsies are recommended when there is some question whether a suspected lesion is of prostate origin or a new primary. Bone scans are reliable if done carefully and serially throughout the patient's clinical disease course. Periodic evaluation of prostate-specific antigen (PSA) levels is helpful in that we currently feel that an elevated value with a positive bone scan is good evidence for recurrence. An X-ray is also helpful, especially if the PSA is normal. In our opinion elevated PSA values alone are not acceptable proof of recurrence. Other correlations should be attempted.

During the course of the NPCP studies, the use of the Gleason Grade for the primary tumour was adopted by many. The limitation of applying such systems to individual cases continues to be overlooked by many physicians. However, the big question: which system, of several, would work best, was in the hands of the pathologist for some time. We evaluated just that and described it in 1986 [5]. The study focus at that time was not survival but progression-free survival. The NPCP

Table 1. TNM Classification 1992: The prostate

T   Primary tumour

Tx   Primary tumour cannot be assessed
T0   No evidence of primary tumour
T1   Clinically unapparent tumour, not palpable nor visible by imaging
         T1a   Tumour an incidental histological finding in 5% or less of tissue resected
         T1b   Tumour an incidental histological finding in more than 5% of tissue resected
         T1c   Tumour identified by needle biopsy (e.g. because of elevated serum PSA)

T2   Tumour confined within the prostate (1)
         T2a   Tumour involves half a lobe or less
         T2b   Tumour involves more than half a lobe but not both lobes
         T2c   Tumour involves both lobes
Note (1) Tumour found in one or both lobes by needle biopsy, but not palpable or visible by imaging, is classified as T1c

T3   Tumour extends through the prostate capsule (2)
         T3a   Unilateral extracapsular extension
         T3b   Bilateral extracapsular extension
         T3c   Tumour invades seminal vesicle(s)
Note (2) Invasion into the prostatic apex or into (but not beyond) the prostatic capsule is not classified as T3 but as T2

T4   Tumour is fixed or invades adjacent structures other than seminal vesicles
         T4a   Tumour invades bladder neck and/or external sphincter and/or rectum
         T4b   Tumour invades levator muscles and/or is fixed to pelvic wall

N   Regional lymph nodes

Nx   Regional lymph nodes cannot be assessed
N0   No regional lymph-node metastasis
N1   Metastasis in a single regional lymph node, 2 cm or less in greatest dimension
N2   Metastasis in a single regional lymph node, more than 2 cm but not more than 5 cm
N3   Metastasis in a regional lymph node more than 5 cm in greatest dimension

M   Distant metastases

Mx   Presence of distant metastasis cannot be assessed
M0   No distant metastasis
M1   Distant metastasis
         M1a   Non-regional lymph node(s)
         M1b   Bone(s)
         M1c   Other site(s)
Note   When more than one site of metastasis is present, the most advanced should be used for staging

---

score (the sum of glandular and nuclear grades) was superior to the previously reported NPCP grade (the maximum of the two grades). The Gleason score was somewhat superior to both NPCP systems [5]. However, this applies only to the primary tumour and not to the nature of any future metastatic lesions. It is clear, however, from our own and other group studies, that the higher the primary tumour score, the more likely pelvic lymph-node involvement would be found when staging lymphadenectomy was performed [6]. Most groups had diffi-

Table 2. NPCP response criteria for objective progression * (any of the following)

1. Significant cancer-related deterioration in weight (>10%), symptoms, or performance status
2. Appearance of new areas of malignant disease
3. Increase in any previously measurable lesion by greater than 25% in cross-sectional area
4. Development of recurring anaemia secondary to prostate cancer - (not treatment-related - Protocols 500[a] and 600[b])
5. Development of ureteral obstruction (Protocols 500[a] and 600[b])

---

* An increase in acid or alkaline phosphatase alone is not to be considered an indication of progression, but should be used in conjunction with other criteria

[a] A comparison of cyclophosphamide (NSC-2671) plus estracyt (NSC-89199) vs cyclophosphamide plus diethylstilboestrol (DES) vs DES or orchidectomy in newly diagnosed patients with clinical stage D cancer of the prostate who had not had prior hormonal therapy, conducted from July 1976 to September 1980

[b] A comparison of diethylstilboestrol (DES) vs DES plus estramustine phosphate in patients with clinical stage D prostatic carcinoma that are stable to hormones or orchidectomy, conducted from July 1976 to present

Table 3. NPCP response criteria for objective complete response (all of the following)

1. Tumour masses, if present, totally disappeared and no new lesions appeared
2. Elevated acid phosphatase, if present, returned to normal
3. Osteolytic lesions, if present, recalcified
4. Osteoblastic lesions, if present, disappeared
5. If hepatomegaly is a significant indicator, there must be a complete return in liver size to normal[a], and normalisation of all pre-treatment abnormalities of liver function, including bilirubin mg%, and SGOT[b]
6. No significant cancer-related deterioration in weight (>10%), symptoms, or performance status

---

[a] Liver size measured by distention below both costal margins at mid-clavicular lines and from the tip of the xiphoid process during quiet respiration without liver movement

[b] SGOT = serum glutamic oxalecetic transaminase

Table 4. NPCP response criteria for objective partial regression (all of the following)

1. At least one tumour mass, if present, was reduced by >50% in cross-sectional area
2. Elevated acid phosphatase, if present, returned to normal
3. Osteolytic lesions, if present, underwent recalcification in one or more, but not necessarily in all
4. Osteoblastic lesions, if present, did not progress
5. If hepatomegaly is a significant indicator, there must be at least a 30% reduction in liver size[a] and at least a 30% improvement of all pre-treatment abnormalities of liver function, including bilirubin mg%, and SGOT[b]
6. There may be no increase in any other lesion and no new areas of malignant disease may appear
7. No significant cancer-related deterioration in weight (>10%), symptoms, or performance status

---

[a] Liver size measured by distention below both costal margins at mid-clavicular lines and from the tip of the xiphoid process during quiet respiration without liver movement

[b] SGOT = serum glutamic oxalecetic transaminase

culty using bone scans to evaluate response to treatment. While individual investigators today continue to promote their own versions, few have stood the test of a multicentre application using quality control and careful checkup procedures. The NPCP established such a success story and reported it [7]. There remains at present no substitute for evaluation of the bony responses. However, using SPET techniques, our new radiolabelled antibody will probably play an important role [4].

In the United States, the only multicentre detection trial, using PSA, ultrasound, and digital rectal examination (DRE) in asymptomatic men, that has reported their results in a peer-reviewed journal has been the one sponsored by the American Cancer Society (ACS) [8]. Based on these results the ACS, together with the American Urological Association and the American College of Radiology, are re-evaluating the ACS guidelines for detection of cancer in asymptomatic persons. One version would recommend, in men 50 years and over, an annual DRE and PSA, and that if either were abnormal further evaluation should be considered.

Table 5. NPCP response criteria for objectively stable disease (all of the following)

---

1. No new lesions occurred and no measurable lesions increased more than 25% in cross-sectional area
2. Elevated acid phosphatase, if present, decreased, though not necessarily returning to normal
3. Osteolytic lesions, if present, did not appear to worsen
4. Osteoblastic lesions, if present, remained stable
5. Hepatomegaly, if present, did not worsen by more than a 30% increase in liver measurements[a] and hepatic abnormalities did not worsen, including bilirubin mg% and SGOT[b]
6. No significant cancer-related deterioration in weight (>10%), symptoms, or performance status

---

[a] Liver size measured by distention below both costal margins at mid-clavicular lines and from the tip of the xiphoid process during quiet respiration without liver movement

[b] SGOT = serum glutamic oxalecetic transaminase

Table 6. Prostate cancer adjuvant study factors

---

1. Primary treatment variables
2. Staging for extent of disease
3. Pathology (primary, secondary, lymph nodes, special tissue studies)
4. Blood test surveillance
5. Interim study (frequency)
6. Other tests for extent of disease, recurrence, metastases
   A. *Blood tests*
   B. *Radioisotope scans*
   C. *Ultrasound*
   D. *CT scan*
   E. *Fine-needle aspiration (cytology)*
   F. *Special tissue studies*
7. Time factors
   A. *Recurrence rate over time*
   B. *Time to recurrence or disease-free interval*
   C. *Survival*

Regardless of the recommendations of individual experts, or even large cooperative groups, what the individual physician does employ determines the cancer control effectiveness of any particular cancer. Early detection has been the hallmark of most efforts. In the United States, since 1976 it has been possible to assess such national responses using the patient care evaluation programme of the Commission on Cancer of the American College of Surgeons (ACOS). This programme, sponsored by the American Cancer Society, uses the tumour registry reports from nearly 2,000 hospitals which reflect from 75-81% of the newly diagnosed cancers seen in the U.S.A. in a given year [9,10]. We have such data for prostate cancer available from 1974-1983 as described [9,10]. In addition, we are now preparing data for another report covering the period 1984-1990 using the ACS/ACOS National Cancer Data Base and the American College of Surgeon's patient care evaluation study. Preliminary data will be herein utilised for this report. From 1974-1983, transurethral resection (TUR) continued to be the most common means to establish the diagnosis of prostatic cancer [9,10]. Over the same time period, nearly 40% of the newly diagnosed prostate cancer patients continued to be in C or D stage and thus not eligible for treatment with a goal of cure. Acid phosphatase and bone scans were more widely used as initial evaluations in the 1980s [9,10]. The measured survival rates did improve.

Let us examine how this has changed in the years 1984-1990, and perhaps project the future. Table 7 summarises the major techniques used for the initial diagnosis of prostate cancer. DRE and TUR remain important measures to detect prostate cancer. A significant change seems to have occurred. The number of cases

Table 7. Preliminary data, American College of Surgeons 1984-1990 National Survey for Prostate Cancer

| | Method of diagnosis | |
	1984	1990
TUR	55.3%	43.0%
Digital rectal examination	54%	53.8%
Needle biopsy	25.1%	26.4%
Transrectal ultrasound biopsy	1.5%	20.6%

(More than one technique may be employed)

using transrectal ultrasound-guided biopsy rose from 1.5% to 20%. Concurrently, in the newly diagnosed cases, PSA utilisation rose from 5.5% to 68% while prostatic acid phosphatase use fell from 62.9% to 50.2%. Clearly, ultrasound (TRUS) and PSA are being employed at the community level in the diagnosis of prostate cancer. The use will likely increase for the foreseeable future. During this same period there was no change in the histological appearance of the newly diagnosed primary tumours. (Well differentiated 26.9%; moderately differentiated 41.0%; poorly differentiated 20.9%; undifferentiated 1.5%; unknown 9.4%; other 0.3%).

With the use of new markers and techniques for early diagnosis, the question remained: Would early state cancers be found? We will therefore review the data on stage found in Table 8.

First, let us deal with the percentage of unknown cases which show a clear increase. Based on other data, this percentage equally affects all clinical stages and not C or D alone. It does reflect an increase in unstaged or unknown data cases. This is clearly a problem in the United States and is being addressed. There is a general trend for a decrease in advanced cases declining over time, with the most marked decline occurring from 1984-1990 when PSA and TRUS biopsy were on an increase. Both measures seem to be associated with this event. Physicians staged 84.4% of all new cases in 1984 and 80% in 1900, so there has been no significant change.

The treatment changes of prostate cancer also reflect the earlier stages of disease being diagnosed, as shown in Table 9. Clearly, the numbers of TURs have dropped and the number of prostatectomies doubled. The majority of the latter are performed retropubically.

Very few cases seen in 1984-1990 were entered on a protocol, either in-house or cooperative group, for radiation or surgical study (1984 1.5%, 1990 1.9%). Cases put on protocol are generally better evaluated, including the stage, compared to those that are not. These few cases on study also reflect the lack of resources now nationally available for clinical trials of prostate cancer in the United States.

The types of treatment for metastatic cancer have also dramatically changed from 1984 to 1990, as shown in Table 10. Oestrogen use fell while antiandrogens rose. Orchidectomy

Table 8. Clinical stage at diagnosis for new prostate cancer cases seen in National American College of Surgeons survey

	1974	1983	1984	1990
Clinical stage				
C	19.3%	13.3%	10.8%	10.2%
D	23.4%	26.5%	27.1%	23.3%
Subtotal	42.7%	39.8%	37.9%	33.5%
Unknown	9.2%	7.6%	14.7%	19.0%

Table 9. Preliminary data, American College of Surgeons 1984-1990 national survey for prostate cancer

Type of primary treatment	1984	1990
TURP	56.7%	41.1%
Prostatectomy	12.0%	24.8%

Table 10. Preliminary data, American College of Surgeons 1984-1990 national survey for prostate cancer

Type of hormones administered for treatment of metastatic cancer	1984	1990
Oestrogen	55.9%	14.3%
Antiandrogens	0.8%	17.0%
Progestational agents	0.6%	0.7%
Orchidectomy	51.4%	66.9%
Other	1.8%	2.3%

(Some cases may have more than one agent for initial treatment)

was the more common treatment in 1990. This is rather surprising in light of the many trials using combined androgen blockade. During this same time period, there was no detectable change in the techniques used to detect recurrence or progression of disease. Additional studies in the future will be necessary to detect the changing role in the U.S.A. for PSA. In conclusion, all the available data we have at hand, based on national surveys in the United States, confirm that PSA and TRUS are being widely employed to diagnose prostate cancer. Concurrently, the clinical stages of the cancers are more often localised and more readily available for primary treatment. The number of prostatectomies performed has doubled in the last 6 years of these studies. Orchidectomy remains a common treatment for advanced disease, despite the introduction of combined androgen blockade protocols. Studies in the future, after 1990, will be necessary for further conclusions.

Additional data from the current era must be completed before any comments could be made regarding other therapies. The main issue for the future, based on theses data, will be which cancers found at an early stage require which treatment, and is it appropriate to only follow certain cancers. The further definition of at risk populations, beyond race or age, is underway and may influence future recommendations for detection, follow-up, and staging.

REFERENCES

1   Murphy GP, Slack NH: Response criteria for the prostate, of the USA National Prostatic Cancer Project. The Prostate 1980 (1):375-382
2   Murphy GP: Markers of prostatic carcinoma. Arch Surg 1991 (26):1404-1407
3   Horoszewicz JS, Murphy GP: Prospective new developments in laboratory research and clinical trials in prostatic cancer. Cancer (supplement) 1990 (66):1083-1085
4   Wynant CE, Murphy GP, Horoszewicz JS, Neal CE, Collier BD, Mitchell E, Purnell G, Tyson I, Heal A, Abdel-Nab H, Winzelberg G: Immunoscintigraphy of prostatic cancer: preliminary results with ^{111}In-labelled monoclonal antibody 7E11-C5.3 (CYT-356). The Prostate 1991 (18):229-241
5   Gaeta JF, Englander LC, Murphy GP: Comparative evaluation of national prostatic cancer treatment group and Gleason systems for pathologic grading of primary prostatic cancer. Urology 1986 (27):306-308
6   Murphy GP: Staging and grading of prostate cancer. Urology Times 1981 (9):10-12
7   Slack NH, Karr JP, Chu TM, Murphy GP: An assessment of bone scans for monitoring osseous metastases in patients being treated for prostate carcinoma. The Prostate 1980 (1):259-270
8   Mettlin C, Lee F, Drago J, Murphy GP: The American Cancer Society National Prostate Cancer Detection Project. Cancer 1991 (67):2949-2958
9   Murphy GP, Natarajan N, Pontes JE, Schmitz RL, Smart CP, Schmidt JD, Mettlin C: The national survey of prostate cancer in the United States by the American College of Surgeons. J Urol 1982 (127):928-934
10 Schmidt JP, Mettlin CJ, Natarajan N, Peace BB, Beart RW Jr, Winchester DP, Murphy GP: Trends in patterns of care for prostatic cancer 1974-1983: results of surveys by the American College of Surgeons. J Urol 1986 (136):416-421

Radical Prostatectomy

Patrick C. Walsh

James Buchanan Brady Urological Institute, Johns Hopkins Medical Institutions, Baltimore, Maryland 21287-2101, U.S.A.

Radical prostatectomy is the oldest continuously employed treatment for prostate cancer. The technique of radical perineal prostatectomy was developed by Hugh Hampton Young at The Johns Hopkins Hospital in 1904. Since that time a variety of therapeutic alternatives have become available: transurethral resection for the relief of bladder outlet obstruction, hormonal therapy and radiation therapy. With the development of these therapeutic alternatives and with a greater understanding of the limitations of radical surgery in the cure of prostatic cancer, it has become necessary on many occasions to redefine the criteria for the selection of surgical candidates. Simply stated, to cure carcinoma of the prostate with surgery the tumour must be confined to the prostate and all tumour must be removed. In the past, few patients were felt to be candidates for surgery because most men presented with advanced stages of the disease and the side effects of surgery were felt by many to be worse than the disease.

Today, the situation is different. With the application of routine digital rectal examination, sequential measurements of prostate-specific antigen (PSA), and improved techniques for outpatient biopsy of the prostate with or without ultrasound guidance, more men present with early stage disease. Also, with improved surgical techniques which have reduced morbidity, radical prostatectomy can be offered to patients with less fear of side effects. Together, these factors have increased the number of patients who are candidates for surgery. However, at the same time, new problems have been introduced into the equation. There are many older patients who are diagnosed with early stage disease. How should they be treated? Also, as in the past, there are still patients who are diagnosed at a time when

it is uncertain whether their disease can be cured. Should they be offered surgery?

For these reasons, it is important to return to the principles of the past. Radical prostatectomy is indicated for the cure of prostate cancer in patients who will live long enough to benefit. For patients who are too old, too ill, or have disease too far advanced, the major principle in management should be palliation of symptomatic disease.

This chapter will review the selection of candidates, surgical technique, results, complications, and prospects for the future.

Selection of Surgical Candidates

First and foremost, the patient should be young and healthy enough to have a 10-15 year life expectancy (Table 1). Studies of conservative therapy of men who presented with localised prostatic cancer have demonstrated that 75% will develop progression and 13-20% will die of their disease during the first 10 years after diagnosis. Thus, although many patients may require hormonal therapy or radiation therapy for palliation, radical prostatectomy is not necessary for men with a life expectancy shorter than one decade.

For patients who are young and healthy, the next question is whether the disease has been detected at a time when cure is possible. This assessment requires a careful physical examination to determine accurately the stage of the local lesion, a review of the histology by an experienced pathologist, a bone scan, and measurement of serum enzymatic acid phosphatase and PSA. In patients who appear to have localised prostatic cancer, it is my experi-

Table 1. Indications for radical prostatectomy

- Cure of prostate cancer in men who will live long enough to benefit

- Candidates:

    T1a - age < 60 years; PSA > 1 ng/ml

    T1b, T1c (selected)

    T2 - Gleason score plus PSA

    T3 - ?; no hormonal downstaging; young men

---

ence that transrectal ultrasound, computed tomography and magnetic resonance imaging (MRI) do not provide additional information that is reliable. However, it is possible that the use of endorectal surface coils in the future may improve the accuracy of MRI. Today, because only 5-10% of men who are felt to be suitable for radical prostatectomy will turn out to have positive lymph nodes, laparoscopic pelvic lymph node dissection appears unnecessary and potentially harmful.

The ideal candidates for radical prostatectomy are patients with T1 or T2 disease. Patients with T1a disease deserve special comment. Although 90% of men with T1a disease will have residual tumour following their initial transurethral resection of the prostate, only about 16% of these patients develop progression over the next 10 years. Recognising that it may be possible to follow these patients with sequential PSA measurements and treat only at the time of progression, there is still controversy about which patient with T1a disease is a candidate for radical prostatectomy. We reserve initial surgical therapy for those patients who are under age 60 and have a post-prostatectomy PSA >1 ng/ml.

For other T1 and T2 patients, the combination of digital rectal examination, Gleason score, and PSA is very useful in determining which patients are likely to have organ-confined disease and benefit most from radical prostatectomy. Because the expression of PSA is inversely related to the Gleason score (e.g. more poorly differentiated tumours produced less PSA per gram of tissue), one must know both the Gleason score and PSA to predict pathologic stage. For example, for a patient with stage T2b disease and a PSA <4 ng/ml, the likelihood

of having organ-confined cancer is 67% if his tumour is a Gleason 5 and 31% if it is a Gleason 8. For the same patient with stage T2b disease and a PSA 4-10 ng/ml, the likelihood of having organ-confined cancer is 56% if he has Gleason 5 disease and 20% if he has Gleason 8 disease. Regardless of Gleason score, in patients with T2b disease who present with PSA levels of 20 ng/ml or greater, the likelihood of organ-confined disease is 1-11%.

Patients with clinical stage T3 disease are not ideal candidates for radical prostatectomy. However, in a small number of patients with low-grade disease who have minimal extension beyond the prostate, cure is possible. Thus, young men who fall into this category may be considered candidates for radical prostatectomy. I do not believe in the use of preoperative hormonal therapy to "downstage" lesions to make them resectable. This has never made sense to me because androgen insensitive tumour cells must exist beyond the boundaries of resection and most certainly will result in treatment failure.

Given these estimations of pathologic stage, the clinician must integrate this with the age of the patient. If the odds for organ-confined disease are not good and the patient is older, he should be encouraged to pursue palliation with external beam radiotherapy or hormonal treatment. In young patients, however, it seems reasonable to offer radical prostatectomy even if the chances for organ-confined cancer are not that great. Using modern surgical techniques, the morbidity of radical prostatectomy today is similar to external beam radiotherapy and many young patients want the chance to be cured.

Surgical Technique

Radical Retropubic Prostatectomy

Over the past 15 years an anatomical approach to radical prostatectomy has been developed for the treatment of localised prostate cancer (Table 2). This procedure emphasises the principle of direct intraoperative visualisation and identification of the exact extent of disease with wide excision where necessary. Delineation of the anatomy of the dorsal vein complex enables the procedure to be per-

Table 2. Anatomical radical prostatectomy: historical development

Year	Anatomy/Technique	Impact
1976	Anatomy of dorsal vein complex and surgical control	Reduced blood loss; Improved visualization
1982	Anatomy of pelvic plexus and identification of cavernous nerves	Nerve-sparing; Preservation of potency
1984	Wide excision of neurovascular bundle	Improved surgical margins
1986	Eversion of bladder neck mucosa	Reduced bladder neck contractures
1989	Anatomy of the striated sphincter	Improved continence

formed in a bloodless field and identification of the anatomy of the pelvic plexus has made it possible to preserve sexual function in most men. This procedure has been developed based upon sound anatomical and pathological principles: 1) the autonomic branches of the pelvic plexus to the corpora cavernosa are located outside the capsule of the prostate and Denonvilliers' fascia; and 2) delineation of the anatomy of the cavernous nerves and their relationship to the capsular arteries and veins of the prostate (neurovascular bundle) and prostatic fascia has made it possible to obtain a wider margin of resection than was previously possible by blunt dissection. It must be emphasised that previously during radical perineal prostatectomy or standard radical retropubic prostatectomy the neurovascular bundles were not routinely resected. Rather, they were inadvertently stretched or torn during these procedures because their existence and significance was not appreciated. Some urologists, however, have criticised the "nerve-sparing technique" because of concern that preservation of potency may compromise cancer control. It is imperative to understand that nerve-sparing is only one technique in an anatomical approach to radical prostatectomy; the converse is wide excision. In fact, by knowing the location of the neurovascular bundles, the surgeon can obtain wider margins by excising this tissue when necessary to remove all tumour. With reduced blood loss and with improved understanding of the striated sphincter, it is also possible to perform a more precise apical dissection to avoid injury to the pelvic floor musculature and

to achieve an accurate sutured vesicourethral anastomosis with coaptation of the mucosal surfaces. This has reduced the frequency of postoperative incontinence.

Radical Perineal Prostatectomy

Radical perineal prostatectomy offers advantages over the retropubic approach: 1) there is less blood loss because the prostate is removed inside the lateral pelvic fascia and Santorini's plexus; 2) the urethra is more easily visualised via the perineal route facilitating the anastomosis; and 3) if the likelihood of pelvic lymph nodes is low or a laparoscopic lymph node dissection is performed, the patient is spared an abdominal incision. On the other hand, because the dissection is performed inside the lateral pelvic fascia, the prostate is more or less enucleated from the surrounding soft tissue and wide margins of excision cannot be achieved. Furthermore, it is difficult to identify the neurovascular bundles via the perineal route, thus making preservation of potency less certain.

Results

The principal goal of radical prostatectomy is cure. Over the past 90 years the definition of cure has undergone continuous refinement. Originally, Hugh Young felt he had cured the

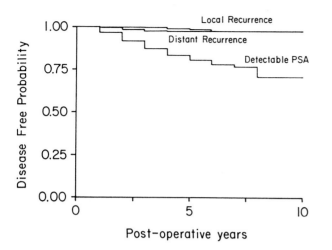

Fig. 1. Actuarial status of 953 consecutive men with clinical stage A and B adenocarcinoma of the prostate who underwent anatomical radical prostatectomy between the years 1982 and 1991

disease if the patient lived for 5 years. Subsequently, Hugh Jewett provided a scholarly critical analysis of the results of radical prostatectomy and stated that tumour-free survival for 15 years or more should be established as the practical yardstick for comparison with other therapeutic methods. However, this included death from all causes and during a 15-year followup fewer men with localised disease die of prostate cancer than of other causes. For this reason, cause-specific actuarial survival analyses are necessary. These analyses focus on the impact of a disease process on survival, since men dying from causes unrelated to carcinoma of the prostate are considered lost to follow-up as of date of death. This statistical assumption is valid when the probability of a non-cancer death is independent of the probability of a cancer death. Using cause-specific criteria, the likelihood of a patient with stage B1 disease dying of prostate cancer over 15 years is 14%.

More recently, earlier endpoints rather than death have been used as indicators of first sign of failure: local recurrence, distant metastases, and elevation of serum PSA (the most sensitive criterion). Using these endpoints, we have recently analysed 953 consecutive men with clinical stage A and B disease who underwent anatomical radical prostatectomy at The Johns Hopkins Hospital in the interval 1982-1991 (Table 3). The tumour was confined to the prostate in 37%, there was focal capsu-

Table 3. Actuarial status of 953 stage A and B men who underwent anatomical radical prostatectomy 1982-1991

Clinical stage

T1a	5%
T1b	10%
T1c	2%
T2	83%

Pathological stage

Organ confined: 37%
Focal capsular penetration: 20%
Established capsular penetration: 28%
Seminal vesicle involvement: 7%
Lymph node involvement: 8%

Follow-up

Median: 4 years
Longer than 8 years: 100 men

Actuarial status at 8 years

Local recurrence: 4%
Distant metastases: 3%
Elevated PSA alone: 35%

lar penetration in 20%, there was extensive capsular penetration in 28%, there was seminal vesicle involvement in 7% and lymph-node involvement in 8%. The median follow-up is 4 years; 100 men have been followed 8 years or longer. At 8 years, 4% had local recurrence, 7% developed distant metastases, and 23% of the men had an elevated PSA alone (Fig. 1). In men with organ-confined cancer, 90% had undetectable levels of PSA. In men with positive seminal vesicles or positive lymph nodes, virtually all had elevated PSA levels. Capsular penetration in the absence of seminal vesicle or lymph-node involvement was present in 48% of the patients. In patients with negative surgical margins and Gleason 2-6 scores, no significant progression was seen. In patients with positive surgical margins and Gleason 2-6 disease or in patients with negative surgical margins but Gleason 7-10 disease, approximately 50% developed an elevated PSA by 8 years. In patients with positive surgical margins and Gleason 7-10 disease, approximately 70% developed an elevated PSA by 8 years. In this series adjuvant postoperative radiotherapy was not employed. When patients with an isolated elevation of PSA underwent delayed radiation therapy, PSA fell to the undetectable range in 15%. Whether immediate adjuvant radiotherapy would have improved on these overall results is unknown.

These data indicate that radical prostatectomy cures the vast majority of men with organ-confined tumours or with well to moderately well differentiated tumours that have penetrated the prostatic capsule to the extent where it is possible to obtain a clear surgical margin. In men with capsular penetration and high-grade tumours, about 50% will be cured. Cure is rarely achieved, if ever, in the presence of positive seminal vesicles or positive lymph nodes. Consequently, every effort must be exercised preoperatively to exclude high-stage disease.

The impact of nerve-sparing on cancer control was evaluated in 503 consecutive potent men who underwent surgery between 1982 and 1988. When patients with single positive margins were evaluated, positive margins produced by preservation of the neurovascular bundle were present in 25 (5%) of the cases. These patients have been followed 4-10 years (median 5 years). One man (0.2%) has developed local recurrence and 6 (1.2%) have an elevated PSA as the only sign of failure. Thus at most, 1.4% of men may have been disadvantaged by attempts at preservation of the neurovascular bundle.

Complications

Urinary Continence

Urinary continence following an anatomical approach to radical prostatectomy has been evaluated in 593 consecutive patients. Complete urinary control was achieved in 92% (547/593). Stress incontinence was present in 8% (46/593); 6% (34) wore 1 or fewer pads per day; stress incontinence was sufficient to require placement of an artificial sphincter in 0.3% [2]. No patient was totally incontinent. Age, weight of the prostate, prior transurethral resection of the prostate, pathological stage, and preservation or wide excision of the neurovascular bundles had no significant influence on preservation of urinary control. These data suggest that anatomical factors rather than preservation of autonomic innervation may be responsible for the improved urinary control associated with an anatomical approach to radical prostatectomy.

It is clear that the distal urethral sphincter mechanism is capable of maintaining passive urinary control in most but not all men. For the 8% of men where it is not sufficient, attempts at reconstruction of the bladder neck to provide an additional continence mechanism should be considered.

Sexual Function

Between 1982 and 1988, 600 men aged 34 to 72 years underwent radical retropubic prostatectomy for prostate cancer. Of the 503 patients who were potent preoperatively and followed for a minimum of 18 months, 342 (68%) are potent postoperatively. Three factors were identified that correlated with the return of sexual function: age, clinical and pathologic stage, and surgical technique (preservation or excision of the neurovascular bundle). In men under 50, potency was similar in patients who had both neurovascular bundles preserved and patients who had 1 neurovascular bundle widely excised (Table 4). With advancing age over 50 years sexual function was better in patients in whom both neurovascular bundles were preserved than in patients in whom 1 neurovascular bundle was excised (p <0.05). When the relative risk of postoperative impotence was adjusted for age, the risk of postoperative impotence was 2-fold greater if there was capsular penetration or seminal vesicle invasion or if one neurovascular bundle was excised (p <0.05).

These data indicate that the return of sexual function postoperatively in men over age 50 years is quantitatively related to preservation of autonomic innervation. In these men where it is necessary to excise the neurovascular bundle on one side, consideration in the future should be given to approaches that may restore autonomic function through nerve regeneration, e.g., partial excision of the bundle or cavernous nerve grafts.

Table 4. Influence of age, surgical technique and pathological stage on recovery of sexual function

| | Post-operative Potency (%) | | | |
| | Both N.V.B. preserved | | One N.V.B. widely excised | |
Age (years)	Organ confined	Positive SV	Organ confined	Positive SV
<50	91%	-	100%	100%
50-60	79%	100%	71%	50%
60-70	71%	44%	62%	17%
>70	17%	-	0%	0%

NVB = neurovascular bundle; SV = seminal vesicle

Conclusions

Over the past 90 years radical prostatectomy has been used in the treatment of men with localised prostate cancer. Based upon anatomical studies, the surgical technique has undergone a continuous evolution. Almost certainly, there will be further advances in anatomy and physiology that will improve the outcome of patients. At present it is possible to cure most men with organ-confined cancer and many men with specimen-confined tumours. With the ability to perform wide excision of tumours, clinical local recurrence rates are low and most patients who fail do so from distant metastases. To improve upon the ability of radical prostatectomy to cure prostate cancer the disease will have to be diagnosed earlier before it has escaped the prostate or improved techniques for adjuvant chemotherapy or immunotherapy must be developed. Although the morbidity of radical prostatectomy is acceptable, simplified approaches to the management of stress urinary incontinence must be developed for the small minority of patients who develop this significant complication. Furthermore, with improved understanding of the physiology of penile erection, someday it may be possible to preserve or simply restore sexual function in almost every man. With these developments, radical prostatectomy will maintain its well deserved position in the cure of prostatic cancer.

REFERENCES

Personal References

1   Quinlan D, Epstein JI, Carter B and Walsh PC: Sexual function following radical prostatectomy: Influence of preservation of neurovascular bundles. J Urol 1991 (145):998- 1002
2   Morton RA, Steiner MS and Walsh PC: Cancer control following anatomical radical prostatectomy: An interim report. J Urol 1991 (145):1197-1200
3   Walsh, PC: Radical retropubic prostatectomy. In: Walsh PC, Retik AB, Stamey TA and Vaughan ED Jr (eds) Campbell's Textbook of Urology, 6th Edition. WB Saunders, Philadelphia 1992, Vol 3 pp 2865-2864

General References

1   Young HH: The cure of cancer of the prostate by radical perineal prostatectomy (prostato-seminal vesiculectomy): history, literature, and statistics of Young's operation. J Urol 1945 (53):188-256
2   Jewett HJ: The present status of radical prostatectomy for stage A and B prostatic cancer. Urol Clin North Am 1975 (2):105-124
3   Bosch RJHH, Kurth KH and Schroeder FH: Surgical treatment of locally advanced (T3) prostatic carcinoma: early results. J Urol 1987 (138):816-822

Radiation Therapy of Prostate Cancer at Stanford University: An Experience of 36 Years

Malcolm A. Bagshaw and Steven L. Hancock

Stanford University School of Medicine, Department of Radiation Oncology, Stanford, CA 94305, U.S.A.

Radiotherapy for prostatic cancer was started in 1910 by Paschkis and Tittinger in Austria who used a radium source attached to a cystoscope. At about the same time Pasteau in France irradiated the prostate with a radium source carried within a urethral catheter. These techniques were brought to the U.S. between 1915 and 1920 by Hugh Young at Johns Hopkins, Barringer at Memorial Hospital in New York and Bumpus at the Mayo Clinic. Our interest at Stanford was stimulated most directly by the successful reports of Rubin Flocks who, in the early 1950s, injected radioactive colloidal gold (^{192}Au) solutions directly into the prostate and regional lymph nodes. By then, it had been generally conceded that androgen deprivation was palliative, even though initially Huggins had thought it would be curative. Radical prostatectomy, both perineal and retropubic, while well developed, was not widely used for two significant reasons. It almost always induced sexual impotence and the criteria for the selection of patients for radical prostatectomy were not well understood.

In the mid 1960s, Jewett clarified the criteria for surgical resection with his classic articles on the prostate nodule. Today resectability criteria are still undergoing revision, but we believe they are still not sufficiently rigorous, mainly because many urologists have relaxed Jewett's strict requirements regarding the solitary nodule. Most authors who have addressed the problem have found, on the average, a 40% incidence of understaging, or transection of tumour when the surgical specimen is carefully prepared. Furthermore, those authors who have followed patients in whom some degree of transection was discovered have found an approx. 50% reduction in anticipated survival when the surgical margins had been violated by tumour. The problem of post-resection impotence has been reduced by the anatomic dissection introduced by Walsh, but it has not been entirely eliminated.

Early Stanford Experience

In 1955, Kaplan and Ginzton introduced a small linear accelerator for radiation therapy at Stanford University. This was the first linear accelerator in the western hemisphere to be used routinely for radiation treatment, although several were already operational in Britain. The Stanford medical linear accelerator produced a photon beam at an energy of between 4 and 6 MV. It was a little more penetrating than Cobalt 60 teletherapy units and had a sharper penumbra. Later, commercial units produced photon beams with a substantially improved penumbra mainly because the electron focal spot on the photon production target was greatly reduced in diameter. Also, the beam collimators were greatly improved. The original Stanford accelerator was mounted in a commercial Van de Graaff gantry which was suspended from the ceiling. The treatment beam could be inclined from the horizontal to about 45° above the horizontal and declinated from horizontal to vertical. The original design did not permit extraction of electrons but this feature was added later, especially for the treatment of mycosis fungoides and other cutaneous malignancies.

The first prostate treatments at Stanford were given by the senior author in 1956. The first patient was referred by Dr. James Ownby, a senior San Francisco urologist, who had previously treated patients with prostate cancer with an intracavitary radium source placed within a catheter within the prostatic urethra (the Pasteau technique). We believe this was learned by Ownby at Johns Hopkins from his mentor, Hugh Young. The first patient was treated with full 360° rotation with a small beam cross-section of 6x6 cm. Rotational therapy was achieved by immobilising the patient in the standing position on a motor driven rotating platform. Even though Ownby's patient had previously received irradiation by the intracavitary radium source, the treatment seemed to be successful and the next 306 patients were treated in a similar manner for the next 14 years.

During the early 1970s, interest shifted to treatment of the regional lymph nodes as well as to the primary prostatic neoplasm, and by then commercial linear accelerators were available. The original commercial accelerator in the United States was produced by Varian Associates in Palo Alto, CA. It incorporated concepts developed by members of the Stanford radiotherapy group, their radiation physics group and Varian engineers and physicists. The prototype Clinac 6 consisted of a horizontal electron accelerator structure approximately 6 feet in length and 6 inches in diameter, which could be rotated a full 360° around an isocenter. The photon beam exited at 90° to the original electron beam and the central ray of the photon beam passed through the isocenter of rotation. This permitted the patient to be treated in a recumbent position while resting quietly on a cantilevered patient support assembly. The cross-section of the beam was easily shaped by casting individualised heavy metal (cerrobend) beam shaping devices. As the emphasis from the early 1970s was to treat the prostate and the first echelon lymphatic drainage, the shaped multiple fields usually consisted of an anterior and posterior pair and a left and right lateral pair. It was recognised early that in order to reduce untoward side effects, the beam needed to be shaped to protect the posterior wall of the rectum and other vital structures, and that each treatment field should be treated each day. Early in the experience, tumour doses were carried to as high as 8000 rad, but it was soon appreciated that untoward side effects became

unacceptable at this dose. As a result, a total tumour dose of 7000 rad which encompassed the prostate and seminal vesicles was adopted. With the original smaller rotational field, a large number of patients were treated to doses in the 7600 rad range without undue side effects. The current technique has recently been described in detail.

The total Stanford experience presently includes treatment of 1160 patients, as summarised in Table 1. All patients referred for treatment since 1956 are included in the table and the reasons for exclusion from radiotherapy are annotated.

The current status of all patients according to survival, cause-specific survival, freedom from relapse, freedom from local relapse and freedom from distant relapse, is presented in Figures 1-5. Actuarial curves for the various patient groups were calculated by the method of Kaplan and Meier. For these calculations, patients were considered to be at risk from the initial date of radiotherapy. Various actuarial functions are defined as follows:

1) *Survival*: Patients who die of any cause are regarded as failing at the time of death. Living patients are censored at the time of last follow-up and continue in the study.

2) *Cause-specific survival*: Patients who die of prostate cancer are regarded as failing at

Table 1. Stanford University, cancer of the prostate referrals for radiation therapy October 1956-December 31, 1991

Total referrals		2738
Exclusion from analysis		
Consult only	439	
Metastatic disease	743	
Other		
Second primary	97	
Prostatectomy	98	
Unusual primary	6	
Previous XRT	22	
Incomplete XRT	26	
Questionable histology	4	
Implants	89	
Implants + XRT	54	
	————	
	1578	
External beam irradiation only		1160
Disease limited to prostate (DLP)	703	
Extracapsular extension (ECE)	457	

PROSTATIC CANCER

⓪ STAGE T0 (100)   ② STAGE T2 (252)   ④ STAGE T4 (37)

① STAGE T1 (351)   ③ STAGE T3 (420)   ⑥ EXPECTED (1160)

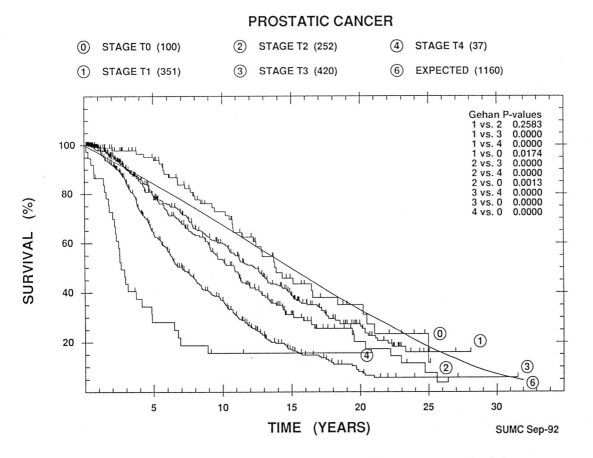

Fig. 1. Survival curves as a function of clinical stage. A downward step represents death from any cause; an upward tick represents a patient surviving at last follow-up and censored at the time indicated by the abscissa. Patient may or may not have residual or metastatic cancer. Number in parentheses is the number of patients in each group.

the time of death. Living patients are censored at the time of last follow-up and patients who die of intercurrent causes are censored at the time of death.

3) *Freedom from relapse*: Patients who relapse either at the primary site or at a metastatic site are regarded as failing at the time of first relapse. Patients who never relapse are censored at the time of last follow-up or intercurrent death.

4) *Freedom from local relapse* (clinical local control): Patients who relapse at the primary site, as determined by clinical examination, are regarded as failing at the time of local relapse. Patients who never relapse locally are censored at the time of last follow-up or death.

5) *Freedom from distant relapse*: Patients who relapse at a metastatic site are regarded as failing at the time of metastatic relapse. Patients whose cancers never metastasize are censored at the time of last follow-up or death.

6) *Expected survival*: The expected survival of a cohort of age-matched American men is plotted as a separate curve in the unabridged survival curves.

The significance of differences between actuarial curves was assessed by the generalised Wilcoxin test of Gehan. Since the lymph node status for most patients was unknown, the lymph node status was ignored. The T-stages according to the Stanford T-Staging System (ST integer)[*] introduced in the early 1970s were utilised in these figures.

---

[*] ST x, 0, 1, 2, 3, 4 denotes Stanford Staging System in the text in order to distinguish it from the AJCC-4 System

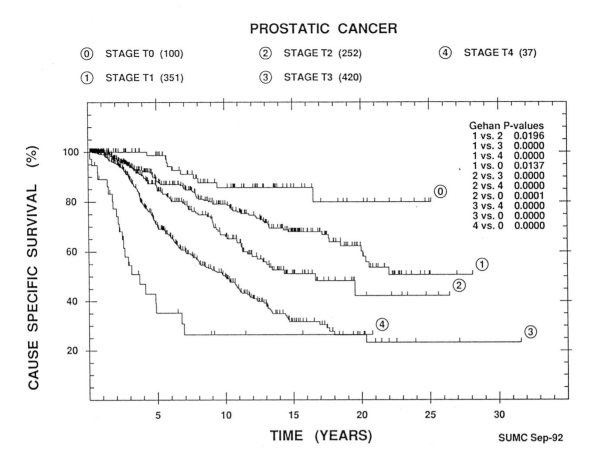

Fig. 2. Cause-specific survival. A downward step indicates death from prostate cancer; an upward tick represents a patient who either died of intercurrent disease without evidence of prostatic cancer or was alive at the time of last follow-up; patient may or may not have had cancer at that time.

Staging

During the development of the Stanford staging system, the patients were first subdivided according to the 12 groupings of the staging system. Actuarial survival curves were generated and Gehan P values were determined for successive pairs of curves. Curves not separated by significant P values were coalesced, which resulted in a family of curves for each endpoint that remarkably, and with only one or two exceptions, grouped the patients into survival patterns that were originally predicted by the T stages. A description of the Stanford ST-staging system is presented in Table 2 along with a comparison with the recently published American Joint Committee, Fourth Edition, Staging System (AJCC-4). The Stanford system has remained unchanged during the past two decades and, by good fortune and a lot of discussion, the AJCC-4 is sufficiently close to it to permit conversion from one to the other.

The only substantial difference is the Stanford ST2 category, which does not exist in either the AJCC-4 or the identical UICC system. Originally, the Stanford ST2 was conceived as an ambiguous category, somewhere between the current AJCC-4/T2 and T3. This encompasses 252 patients who, on initial examination, seemed to fall ambiguously between patients with tumour confined to disease limited by the prostatic capsule (DLP) and to those with extracapsular extension (ECE). We found that it was often difficult to decide between what is now defined as AJCC-4 T2 and T3. Therefore, we created this ambiguous group hoping that time would allow a finer distinction between DLP and ECE. We are not certain the issue has been settled, but the new staging system encourages us to bring the Stanford TNM staging into line with current world opinion. There is, however, one note of concern. As we look at our data on pure survival (Fig. 1), there is no significant difference in survival

Table 2a. Comparison of Stanford-AJCC-4 staging of prostate cancer

Stanford		AJC 4th Edition		Definitions of TNM (AJCC-4th Edition)
TX		TX		Primary tumour cannot be assessed
TX		T0		No evidence of primary tumour
T0		T1		Clinically inapparent tumour not palpable or visible by imaging
	T0f (focal)		T1a	Tumour incidental histological finding in 5% or less of tissue resected
	T0d (diffuse)		T1b	Tumour incidental histological finding in more than 5% of tissue resected
			T1c	Tumour identified by needle biopsy (e.g. because of elevated PSA)
T1		T2		Tumour confined within the prostate*
	T1a)	T2a		Tumour involves half of a lobe or less
	T1b)			
	T1c	T2b		Tumour involves more than half of a lobe, but not both lobes
	T1d	T2c		Tumour involves both lobes
T2		Does not exist		
	T2a	Does not exist		
	T2b	Does not exist		
T3		T3		Tumour extends through the prostatic capsule**
	T3a		T3a	Unilateral extracapsular extension
	T3b		T3b	Bilateral extracapsular extension
	T3b		T3c	Tumour invades the seminal vesicle(s)
T4		T4		Tumour is fixed or invades adjacent structures other than the seminal vesicles
T4			T4a	Tumour invades any of: bladder neck, external sphincter, or rectum
T4			T4b	Tumour invades levator muscles and/or is fixed to the pelvic wall

* Tumour found in one or both lobes by needle biopsy, but not palpable or visible by imaging, is classified as T1c
** Invasion into the prostatic apex or into (but not beyond) the prostatic capsule is not classified as T3, but as T2

Table 2b. Comparison of Stanford, AJCC-4 staging of prostate cancer

AJC 4th Edition		Stanford		Definitions of TNM (Stanford)
TX		TX		Characteristic anatomic relationships distorted and/or absent secondary to major intervention, i.e. suprapubic prostatectomy or prior XRT
T0		TX		No evidence of primary tumour
T1		T0		Occult carcinoma: Incidental finding of carcinoma in the operative specimen
	T1a		T0f (focal)	<5% of specimen
	T1b		T0d (diffuse)	>5% of specimen
	T1c	Does not exist		
T2		T1		Palpable tumour limited by the prostatic capsule without distortion of the superior or lateral anatomic boundaries
	T2a		T1a	Solitary nodule ≤1 cm in diameter with normal, compressible prostatic tissue on 3 sides (lesion amenable to radical prostatectomy)
			T1b	Palpable tumour >1 cm occupying <50% of a lobe
	T2b		T1c	Palpable tumour occupying >50% of a lobe or multiple nodules limited to one lobe
	T2c		T1d	Involvement of both lobes
Does not exist		T2		Palpable tumour of any size primarily limited by the prostatic capsule with minimal distortion of the lateral or superior anatomic boundaries without definite obliteration of a lateral sulcus and/or a seminal vesicle region

Table 2b. Comparison of Stanford, AJCC-4 staging of prostate cancer (contd.)

AJC 4th Edition	Stanford	Definitions of TNM (Stanford)
Does not exist	T2a	Palpable tumour occupying <50% of a lobe
Does not exist	T2b	Palpable tumour occupying >50% of a lobe, multiple nodules limited to one lobe, or involvement of both lobes
T3	T3	Palpable tumour extending beyond the prostatic capsule with definite obliteration of any extent of a lateral sulcus and/or a seminal vesicle region
T3a	T3a	Tumour involving ≤50% of a lobe
T3b	T3b	Palpable tumour occupying ≥50% of a lobe
T3c	T3b	Definite extension into seminal vesicle region
T4	T4	Palpable tumour extending beyond the prostatic capsule with attachment to both pelvic sidewalls, rectal wall invasion, or bladder invasion*
T4a	Not specified	
T4b	Not specified	

*   Patients with IVP findings suggestive of bladder involvement will undergo cystoscopy and biopsy if indicated

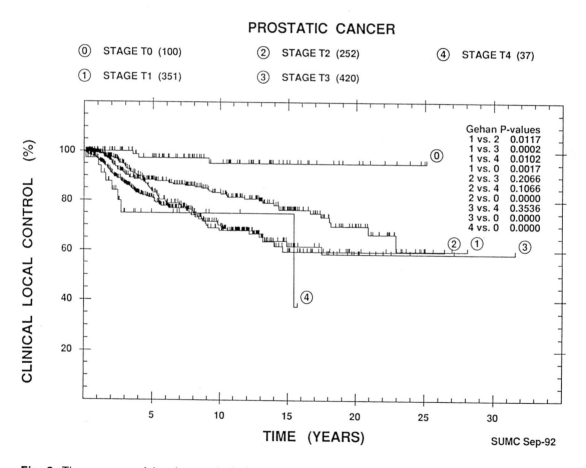

Fig. 3. Time course of local control. A downward step indicates clinical evidence of local regrowth after initial regression of tumour or after an initial showing of no evidence of local neoplasm. An upward tick represents a patient who either demonstrated no clinical evidence of local tumour at last follow-up or died without clinical evidence of local neoplasm. Patient could have had evidence of metastatic tumour either while living or at death. Local control is paradoxically high for stage T4 because many patients die of metastatic disease before lack of local control is manifest.

PROSTATIC CANCER

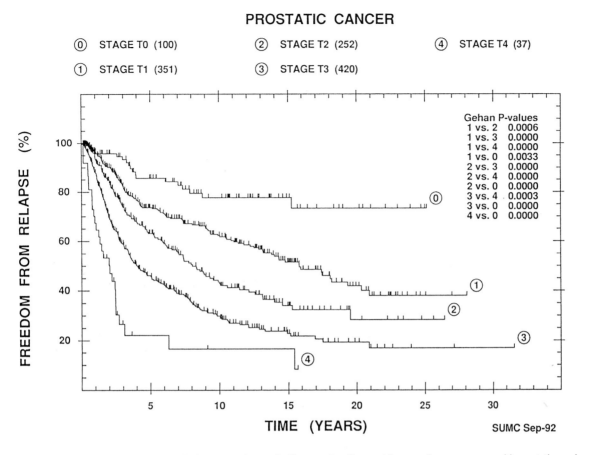

⓪ STAGE T0 (100)   ② STAGE T2 (252)   ④ STAGE T4 (37)

① STAGE T1 (351)   ③ STAGE T3 (420)

Gehan P-values
1 vs. 2 0.0006
1 vs. 3 0.0000
1 vs. 4 0.0000
1 vs. 0 0.0033
2 vs. 3 0.0000
2 vs. 4 0.0000
2 vs. 0 0.0000
3 vs. 4 0.0003
3 vs. 0 0.0000
4 vs. 0 0.0000

SUMC Sep-92

Fig. 4. Freedom from relapse. A downward step indicates the first evidence of recurrence, either at the primary site or at a metastatic site as detected by either clinical observation or by a positive biopsy. An upward tick represents a patient who was either observed disease free or died disease free at the time of last observation.

between our pure DLP group, ST1, and those with possible extracapsular extension, ST2. On the other hand, as we look at cause-specific survival (Fig. 2), there is a clear and highly significant difference between those with well defined disease limited to the prostate, ST1, and those with possible but not definite extracapsular disease, ST3. This may be a key to defining a difference between patients selected for either surgery or radiotherapy. Later in this chapter we will show that there is no difference in survival between our AJCC-4 T1 (ST0) plus AJCC-4 T2a and T2b (ST1 plus some ST2) patients and the expected survival of an age-matched cohort of males (Fig. 7). Our results with radiotherapy appear comparable to short-term results reported for prostatectomy. On the other hand, inspection of Figures 1-5 shows that the long-term results with our ST2 category appear better than generally reported

for nominal B2 or AJCC-4, T2c and some T3 patients. We have long-term follow-up on 252 of these Stanford ST2 patients who fall somewhere between AJCC-4, T2 and T3 patients. We believe our record system and the new AJCC-4 guidelines will permit reallocation of the ST2 patients to the new AJCC-4 system. This work is nearly finished and will be the subject of further research. This will be possible because all patients in the Stanford system were staged by at least two observers. They recorded careful descriptions of the clinical examination of the prostate, with diagrams drawn in all but a few. The author feels comfortable in allocating the Stanford ST2 between the AJCC-4 T2 and T3 categories. (This has now been completed and display of the survival parameters by the AJCC-4 system will be the subject of future publications.)

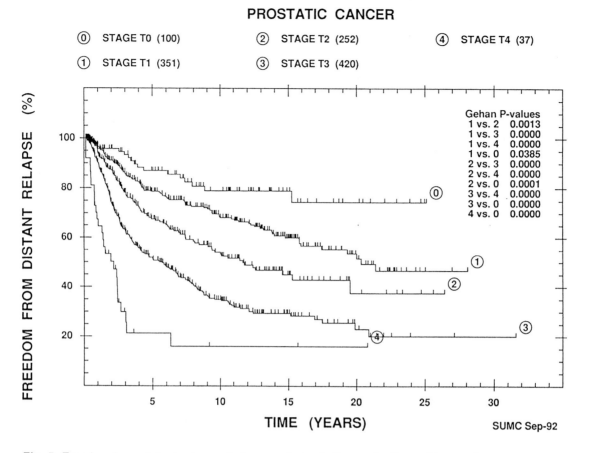

Fig. 5. Freedom from distant relapse. A downward step indicates the first evidence of recurrence at a metastatic site as detected either by clinical observation (including imaging) or a positive biopsy. An upward tick represents a patient who was either observed disease free or died disease free at the time of last observation.

Survival Parameters According to Gleason Score

The Gleason grading system was adopted at Stanford soon after its introduction in the late 1960s. The Stanford pathology department grades the histology by the Gleason system whenever possible; accordingly, 841 of our patients have been scored by the Gleason method. It is interesting that, in terms of survival, the Gleason patterns seem to congregate into 3 groups. Gleason sums of 2,3,4,5 are distinct from either Gleason sums 6 and 7 and also distinct from Gleason sums of 8,9,10. However, there is no statistical difference between Gleason sums 6 and 7 in terms of survival. Figure 6 demonstrates that for cause-specific survival there are 4 distinct groups: Gleason 2,3,4 and 5; Gleason 6; Gleason 7; and Gleason 8,9,10. For clinical local control, there is a different pattern with best clinical local control observed in Gleason sums of 2,3,4,5 +

6 and poor local control for Gleason sums 7 + 8, 9 and 10. Freedom from relapse again is subdivided into 4 distinct groupings whereas, although there is a clear separation between the groups for freedom from distant relapse, again the difference between pattern 6 and 7 is not significant.

Optimal Candidates for Cure (Either Surgery or Radiotherapy)

We define these patients as those with clinically well defined local disease (i.e., low or intermediate stage). Gleason scores were not included as a selection parameter. These patients may also have relatively low but abnormal serum PSA values. This consideration, however, was not available for the evaluation of most of these patients who preceded the advent of the PSA test. These patients could be considered suitable candidates for radical

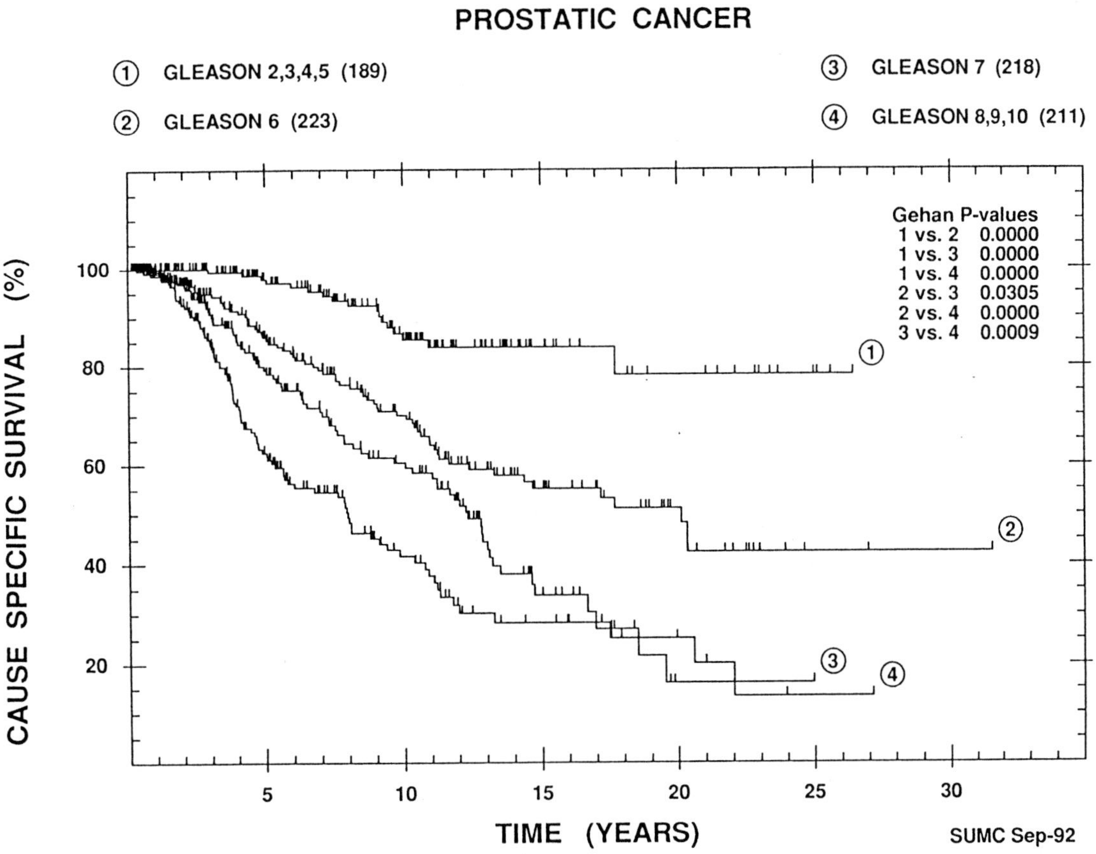
PROSTATIC CANCER
① GLEASON 2,3,4,5 (189)
② GLEASON 6 (223)
③ GLEASON 7 (218)
④ GLEASON 8,9,10 (211)
Gehan P-values
1 vs. 2 0.0000
1 vs. 3 0.0000
1 vs. 4 0.0000
2 vs. 3 0.0305
2 vs. 4 0.0000
3 vs. 4 0.0009
CAUSE SPECIFIC SURVIVAL (%)
100
80
60
40
20
5
10
15
20
25
30
TIME (YEARS)
SUMC Sep-92

Fig. 6. Cause-specific survival as a function of Gleason sum. Note that for cause-specific survival 4 distinctive categories are identified.

resection. They would be found in the Stanford categories ST0, ST1a, ST1b, ST1c. These correspond to the AJCC-4 categories of T1a, T1b, T2a, and T2b. We do not believe patients with bilateral prostate involvement represent good candidates for radical surgery. Nevertheless, it is shown in Figure 1 that patients with Stanford T3, AJCC-4 T3 have a reasonable, albeit diminished chance for cure with irradiation. Patients in the AJCC-4 T1c group also would be considered candidates for radiotherapy or radical surgery. We have not yet broken out this small group of patients, identified only since the advent of the PSA test. In any case, they have been considered within the Stanford ST1a category and included in this group of patients. Survival and cause-specific survival are demonstrated for all 355 patients with ST0, ST1a, ST1b, and ST1c patients (these are and have been identically staged with the AJCC-4 T1a, T1b, T2a, and T2b patients), and there is no significant difference in the observed survival of this group of patients as compared with an age-matched cohort of California males (Fig. 7). The cause-specific survival was 80% at 15 years and 60% at 25 years. It seems inconceivable that in a large group of patients followed for a long period of time any other therapy could produce a better survival record.

Pure survival has been criticised as an inappropriate endpoint to observe in patients with prostatic cancer after any given treatment. It is true that the pressure of intercurrent death in this elderly population may confound the survival endpoint and cause-specific survival has been suggested as superior. We recognised this and reported our disease-specific (cause-specific) survival for these patients in 1987. While we agree that cause-specific survival is a useful parameter, it lacks the specificity of survival only. Prostate patients usually die in their communities, rarely have post-mortem examinations, and the true cause of death is often unknown. In addition to our annual follow-up procedure, we obtain death certificates on de

STANFORD STAGE T0, T1a, T1b, T1c

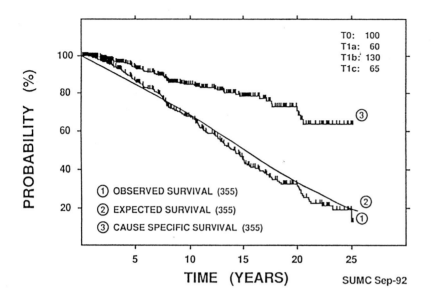

Fig. 7. Stanford stages ST0, ST1a, ST1b and ST1c, curve 1, are compared with the expected survival of an age-matched cohort of Californian males, curve 2. These Stanford stages are essentially identical to the new AJCC-4 definitions for T1a, T1b, T2a and T2b. The AJCC-4 new category T1c has not been segregated but is included with the Stanford T1a group. There are only a few of these patients. Curve 3 details cause-specific survival.

ceased patients. Often it is obvious that the patient died of prostatic cancer, but it is also clear that many patients have death assigned to prostatic cancer simply because at some time they had had the diagnosis. Cause-specific survival, while probably the ideal endpoint, is flawed unless documented by postmortem examination. There is little ambiguity about survival *per se*. Local control is slightly better than 80% at 15 years and 75% at 25 years for this group of optimal patients. Freedom from relapse is 60% at 15 years and 50% at 25 years. Therefore, it appears to us that patients with prostatic cancer confined to at least one lobe of the prostate, who are treated by radiation therapy, have a long-term expectation of survival equivalent to the population at large.

Restaging the Stanford ST2 category is not expected to change significantly the survival pattern for the AJCC-4 T2 patients. It is clear that there will be little change in the survival pattern for this group of patients once they are restaged because a few of the presently classified ST2a patients will be reclassified as AJCC-4 T3a and they will be the least involved stage T3 patients. Whereas when looking at the group of Stanford ST0, ST1a, ST1b, ST1c plus ST2a patients, the few that will be reclassified as AJCC-4 T3 will be removed, presumably improving the survival pattern of that group as well. This is a perfect example of the Will Rogers effect in which a stage shift will likely benefit both new categories. It is already known that the stage shift will be minimal and most likely not statistically significant because approximately one-half of the Stanford ST2 patients have already been reallocated and most of them are falling into the AJCC-4 T2 category.

The fact that some suffer recurrence or metastatic disease cannot be denied. However, this seems to be no different from the outcome reported by Blute et al. in a Mayo Clinic study of 315 patients who had clinically staged localised adenocarcinoma of the prostate confirmed pathologically to be organ confined. In that series, 28 failed locally, 25 failed systemically, and 8 failed both systemically and locally. These failure rates are identical to those seen in a small cohort of the Stanford optimal patients who also had staging laparotomies and lymph nodes proven negative for tumour.

More Advanced Disease

We are not complacent about the present status of radiation treatment of more advanced prostatic cancer. As stage increases, with all that implies such as larger mass of the neoplasm, and poorer cellular differentiation, the probability for successful treatment decreases. We have tried to improve survival in the Stanford ST3, AJCC-4 T3 patients by both increasing the radiation dose and employing adjunctive therapy. We have developed a combination of external beam irradiation, interstitial irradiation, and hyperthermia for the more advanced patients. We have increased the radiation dose by terminating the external beam exposure at 5000 rad in 5 weeks and, after a 2 or 3-week period of rest, adding an interstitial 192-iridium implant which delivers an additional 3000 rad during 60 to 72 hours of inpatient therapy. Metallic trocars are inserted transperineally to facilitate the insertion of the radioactive iridium sources, and these trocars are used to conduct radiofrequency current at 0.5 MHz which elevates the temperature of the prostate to approximately 42.5°C. The hyperthermia treatments are administered for 45 minutes immediately before the insertion of the iridium sources into the conductive interstitial trocars and again after the iridium is removed about 60 hours later just before the trocars are withdrawn. Figure 8 demonstrates our current experience. Clearly, insufficient time has elapsed to evaluate this modality, but to date only 2 patients have had a clinical recurrence. One patient died due to cardiovascular complications, and he had no clinical evidence of persistent cancer. Two additional patients have had post-treatment positive biopsies, but to date have not manifested clinical evidence of either local or metastatic disease. Most patients have not yet been biopsied post-therapy.

Morbidity

Morbidity associated with radiation treatment of prostatic cancer has been dramatically reduced over the past decade as radiotherapists have increasingly employed blocking techniques which confine the radiation closer to the tumour volume. Secondly, they have been more careful to treat multiple fields on a daily basis, which minimises the effects of radiation dose across both time and target tissues.

While it is true that some patients appear to lose sexual potency as a consequence of the radiation, 50% of the patients treated in our series have maintained their sexual potency for a period of 9 years.

Finally, a careful review of new neoplasms in patients treated for prostatic cancer has shown no evidence for the induction of secondary tumours.

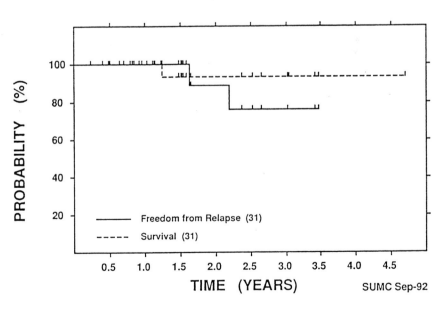

Fig. 8. This demonstrates the current status of patients treated with a combination of external beam irradiation, interstitial implantation by [192] iridium plus hyperthermia

Summary and Conclusions

1)   Treatment of small volume (one lobe or less) prostatic cancer by external beam radiation therapy offers the prospect for long-term survival identical to that enjoyed by the population at large. It is also identical to that for patients who are currently selected for radical prostatectomy.

2)   As tumour stage increases with all that implies, i.e., larger mass of neoplasm and poorer cellular differentiation, the prospect for survival after radiation decreases, but it never reaches zero.

3)   It is not possible to directly compare the outcome for patients treated with surgery vs. radiotherapy as long as clinical staging is subject to nearly 40% error and lymph-node staging is not available for most irradiated patients. On the other hand, clinical staging will improve, probably through the use of transrectal magnetic resonance imaging (MRI), which now can distinguish tumour from normal prostatic tissue and can provide an image of the capsule, permitting, in some cases at least, differentiation of stage AJCC-4 T2 from stage T3. This may promote better case selection between surgery and radiotherapy.

4)   Further improvement in radiotherapy techniques is anticipated by broader use of 3-dimensional treatment planning, and the use of more restricted radiation treatment volumes (conformal therapy).

5)   U.S.A. national trials are in progress to test the efficacy of pre-radiotherapeutic cytoreduction by androgen deprivation and antiandrogens.

6)   Other trials are in progress to test improved efficacy of irradiation by the addition of pharmacological sensitising agents.

7)   Radiosensitisation by hyperthermia appears to have improved our results in patients with more advanced disease.

8)   Radiotherapy is a safe and effective method for the treatment of prostatic cancer. Improved technology in defining the extent of the primary tumour and in the delivery of radiation dose is near at hand. Augmentation of the effectiveness of irradiation by physical and/or pharmacological means seems a promise for the future.

REFERENCES

1   Bagshaw MA, Kaplan HS and Sagerman RH: Linear accelerator supervoltage radiotherapy. VII. Carcinoma of the prostate. Radiology 1965 (85):121-129
2   Bagshaw MA, Cox RS and Ray GR: Status of radiation treatment of prostate cancer at Stanford University. NCI Monographs 1988 (7):47-60
3   Bagshaw MA: Carcinoma of the prostate. In: Levitt SH (ed) Technological Basis of Radiation Therapy: Practical Clinical Applications. Lea & Febiger, 1992 pp 300-322
4   Flocks RH, Kerr HD, Elkins HB and Culp D: Treatment of carcinoma of the prostate by interstitial radiation with radioactive gold (Au^{198}): A preliminary report. J Urol 1952 (68):510-522
5   Hultberg S: Results of treatment with radiotherapy in carcinoma of the prostate. Acta Radiologica 1946 (27):339-350
6   Jewett HJ, Bridge RW, Gray GF Jr et al: The palpable nodule of prostatic cancer. JAMA 1968 (203):403-406

Primary Endocrine Treatment of Advanced Prostate Cancer

Louis J. Denis [1] and Charles Mahler [2]

1 Department of Urology
2 Department of Endocrinology, A.Z. Middelheim and Vrije Universiteit Brussels, Lindendreef 1, 2020 Antwerp, Belgium

Clinical prostate cancer has been recognised as a single biological process with a usually slow but constant growth. This clinical progression can be temporarily arrested by endocrine treatment which offers palliation but will never cure patients with advanced prostatic cancer. Unfortunately, prostate cancer covers a wide range of disease where the biological potential of the tumour predicts prognosis overriding all forms of treatment at any disease stage. It is therefore crucial to incorporate the known and validated prognostic factors into clinical practice so that patients with good prognostic factors may receive the treatment least aggressive to their quality of life, which may even be no treatment, while patients with poor prognostic factors, where survival or the lowest probability of death from prostate cancer is the important endpoint, would be candidates for aggressive treatment.

This state of affairs is likely to create controversies in the management of the disease, leading to errors in treatment by commission or by omission [1]. There is consensus that advanced disease, which usually means metastatic disease, is incurable. This principle can be applied to all stages, from residual tumour after attempts to curative treatment, to widespread metastatic disease detected at first diagnosis with a so-called superscan.

The wide range of disease, the lack of a defined biological potential of the tumour, the number of competing diseases in men at the peak of the incidence of prostate cancer and the variety of endocrine treatment, have led to controversies in the management of advanced prostatic cancer that are not yet resolved. The first step towards successful treatment is, of course, proper diagnosis and staging. The first action after a positive biopsy for prostate cancer, which preferably should be evaluated by the urologist together with the pathologist, is to stage the disease according to the TNM classification and evaluate its prognostic factors [2]. The great majority of metastatic disease with its known predilection to bone is diagnosed by a bone scan. Diffuse back pain, poor performance status and high serum marker levels of prostate specific antigen (PSA) and alkaline phosphatase (ALP) point to the possible diagnosis of bone metastasis. Bone scan and its SPEC derivative are widely used and have replaced all other imaging as the first choice examination. One should remember that this examination is not infallible nor cancer specific and it merely detects metabolically active areas of bone by incorporation of 99 TCM diphosphatase. The reported hot spots are usually controlled by radiography utilising tomography, selected computed tomography or nuclear magnetic resonance. Some localisations such as single skull, cervical vertebrae and shoulder joints should be viewed with caution on a suspect bone scan. Indeed, quality control studies in the trials of the European Organisation for Research and Treatment of Cancer (EORTC) have shown a number of limitations of this procedure in routine clinical use [3].

The confirmed presence of metastatic disease by bone scan and radiography excludes further local or nodal staging procedures. Other routine staging procedures include chest X-ray, liver ultrasound and the usual laboratory tests such as ALP, haemoglobin, creatinine and liver enzymes with PSA as a key indicator of disease activity.

With a negative bone scan, the status of the regional lymph nodes, for prostate cancer the

Table 1. Proposed subdivision of metastatic disease according to the number of foci

M1 disease - Telescopic ramification

Mx	Presence of distant metastasis cannot be assessed		
Mo	No distant metastasis		
M1	Distant metastasis		
	M1a	non-regional lymph node(s)	
	M1b	bone(s)	M1b(I)	metastasis in bone(s), 1-5 foci
			M1B(II)	metastasis in bone(s), 5-20 foci
			M1b(III)	metastasis in bone(s), more than 20 foci or diffuse involvement
	M1c	other site(s)	

pelvic nodes, forms an important prognostic factor. Unfortunately, one needs to proceed to laparoscopic or surgical lymph node dissection to make a diagnosis of lymph node metastasis. Common sense dictates that these interventions are only performed on the indication of a possible curative treatment, which implies radical prostatectomy or radiotherapy.

The incorporation of known and validated prognostic factors is of paramount importance for the selection of appropriate treatment. Total tumour volume is among the most powerful prognostic factors in all stages of the disease including metastatic sites, lymph nodes and primary tumour [4]. The division of M1b (bone) disease according to the number of positive foci has a clear effect on the prognosis [5]. A telescopic ramification of the TNM system has been proposed and its scheme is presented in Table 1. Local tumour extent (T4) and high serum levels of PSA also carry a poor prognosis [6].

Treatment

Treatment selection based on the analysis of prognostic factors has practical life importance as we were able to demonstrate in EORTC study 30853 that the median survival for patients with good prognostic factors was 5.2 years as compared to 2.7 years for patients with intermediate prognostic factors and only 1.6 years for patients with poor prognostic factors. It is clear that definition of these or other related factors provides us with the opportunity to prescribe more individualised treatment [4]. Androgen deprivation in one of its many forms has been the golden standard for treatment of patients with symptomatic advanced disease since the landmark studies of Huggins [7]. The aim of the endocrine treatment is to block cancer cell stimulation by the androgens, resulting in arrest of tumour growth or in tumour regression over a period of time. The treatment results are impressive and show objective remission in 40 to 60% of the patients while 60 to 85% of subjective remissions have been recorded [8]. Since we only institute palliative treatment, we have to consider 5 questions that are relevant to the treatment options and could be discussed with the patients. These questions are listed in Table 2.

Timing of Treatment

Strange though it may seem, there is still debate about the question whether endocrine treatment provides increased survival and is able to influence the natural, untreated history of the disease. Of course the issue under discussion is not that patients do as well without

Table 2. Questions on initial treatment to be discussed with the patient

1. Timing of the treatment ?

2. Indications for this treatment ?

3. Is there a best treatment for response/survival ?

4. Is there a best treatment for the patient ?

5. Neo-adjuvant treatment ?

endocrine treatment, the option concerns treatment timing, that is, immediate initiation at the time of diagnosis or initiation at the occurrence of symptomatic disease. The concept of early versus delayed treatment found its first support in the observations of the Veterans' Administrative Cooperative Urological Research Group (VACURG) trials some 30 years ago; they concluded that hormonal therapy does not influence survival and that 5 mg of diethylstilboestrol (DES) was associated with significant cardiovascular complications and death [9]. Still one cannot fail to note that relapse occurred in 70% of the patients with advanced disease and 100% of the patients with metastatic disease in the follow-up period. A later review of the results concluded that younger patients with undifferentiated tumours and metastatic disease benefit from early hormonal treatment for a minimum follow-up of 36 months [10]. These observations where confirmed in elderly men from a defined geographical area in Sweden with advanced localised prostate cancer. After exclusion of moderately and poorly differentiated cancer, they received essentially expectant treatment consisting of delayed endocrine treatment as 67% of the participants showed disease progression over 5 years [11]. A second confirming phase II study from Sweden emphasised the notion that some localised prostatic cancers in elderly men could be treated expectantly, resulting in a "specific prostate cancer mortality" of only 10% while most of the patients died from other causes [12]. An ongoing randomised trial in Sweden comparing radical prostatectomy versus expectant treatment will hopefully solve this burning question by the year 2000. Two major randomised trials of the Medical Research Council (MRC) and the EORTC specifically address the issue of early versus delayed treatment in patients with asymptomatic metastatic disease. While awaiting the outcome of these trials, one has to realise that there are patients with asymptomatic disease with slowly growing tumours who will never suffer from their cancer or will never benefit from endocrine treatment due to the simple fact that competing causes of death in their age group do not provide the time to suffer or to benefit. Still, in the more recent EORTC trials 30805 and 30853 a full 80% of the patients died by and not with prostatic cancer, with a mean survival of only 2.7 years. However, in the latter trial we were able to show a substantial advantage in time to subjective/objective relapse and even survival by cancer death just by comparing two different endocrine treatments [13].

We expect that all of the ongoing trials will demonstrate that endocrine treatment shifts the survival curve to the right and that the achievement of palliation resulting in quality-of-life benefit over a period of time could or should be the endpoint when treating patients with advanced prostate cancer.

Indications for Endocrine Treatment

The lack of conclusive data on survival benefit is important but merely rethorical since, as stated before, the great majority of patients either receive endocrine treatment at a later stage of disease because symptoms occur or they die of competing diseases. There is consensus that endocrine treatment shows a straightforward subjective and objective response benefit in symptomatic patients as demonstrated by all the endocrine treatment phase II and phase III studies since the landmark demonstration of Huggins [7].

Is There a Best Treatment for Response/Survival?

The available and routinely used first-line treatment options for prostate cancer are presented in Table 3.

There are essentially 3 principles of treatment: androgen withdrawal, androgen blockade and the combination of both treatments called combination treatment or maximal androgen blockade treatment (MAB).

Bilateral Orchidectomy

The elimination of testicular androgens by surgical castration or DES at daily doses of 1 to 5 mg has been regarded as the standard treatment for prostate cancer for 4 decades. The aim of reducing the circulating serum levels of testosterone (T) by surgical castration is easily attained since the procedure removes the circu-

Table 3. Array of current first-line endocrine treatments utilised in daily practice to palliate prostate cancer

Androgen withdrawal

1. Surgical castration: bilateral orchidectomy
                                 subcapsular orchidectomy
                                 subepididymal orchidectomy

2. Medical castration: oestrogens
                                 diethylstilboestrol 1-3 mg/day
                                 polyoestradiol phosphate i.m. 160 mg/month
                                 estramustine phosphate 560 mg/day

                                 LHRH A depot preparations

Androgen blockade

Anti-androgens: cyproterone acetate 300 mg/day

                                 flutamide   750 mg/day*
                                 nilutamide   300 mg/day
                                 casodex   100 mg/day*

Combination treatment

Maximal androgen blockade: LHRH A - anti-androgen
                                 orchidectomy - anti-androgen

* monotherapy clinical research

lating testicular androgens. The complications of the procedure are minimal and the side-effects are associated with androgen withdrawal, resulting in 30 to 40% of the patients complaining of hot flushes. Compliance is, of course, complete and this gives the procedure an edge in all debilitated patients with serious symptoms. For younger patients, the surgical mutilation is harder to accept and when given a choice most patients prefer medical castration [14]. The burden of mutilation can be decreased by performing a subcapsular or a subepididymal orchidectomy [15]. The rapid drop in circulating androgens makes surgical castration one of the best choices in patients with the impending complication of paralysis by metastatic disease.

Oestrogens

Oestrogens cause medical castration by their influence on the negative feedback on the hypothalamo-pituitary gonal axis which results in reduced LH secretion and testicular T synthe-sis. Occasionally, they raise the sex hormone binding globulin levels (SHBG), the plasma prolactin (PRL) levels and direct interaction on prostatic tissue and testis has been demonstrated in experimental work. A dose of 5 mg of DES results in an effective medical castration in the great majority of patients. However, this dose was abandoned since the VACURG studies linked the 5 mg dose to an excessive number of cardiovascular complications and death while the 1 mg dose in later studies proved to be just as effective [10]. Indeed, the efficacy of 1 mg DES was demonstrated in the EORTC 30805 trial where no difference in survival and progression-free survival was noted between 3 arms of a randomised trial comparing bilateral orchidectomy with and without cyproterone acetate versus 1 mg of DES [16]. The non-lethal cardiovascular side-effects for this 1 mg dose were significant but only for leg oedema and dyspnoea, without showing the previously reported lethal complications attributed to DES. These clinical results are remarkable in that it is known that 1 mg of DES brought serum T levels to castrate levels in only 80% of the patients. A further reduction of the dose was not practical since earlier VACURG studies had proven that 0.2 mg of DES was not effective [10]. Efforts to circumvent the cardiovascular risk from oestrogen treatment were made by administering parenteral depot injections of polyoestradiolphosphate [17]. Progesterone derivatives have been reported to be an effective treatment, but the lack of efficiency of a single 250 mg dose a day in EORTC 30761, as well as the absence of their marketing in Europe and the popularity of cyproterone acetate serving simultaneously as a steroid anti-androgen, diminished the interest and the use of the pure progestagens in the treatment of prostate cancer.

The classic combination of estramustine phosphate, widely prescribed for patients with poor prognostic factors, received renewed interest with the demonstration of its clinical activity by binding protein affecting the macrotubular activity of prostate cancer cells and stabilising the disease [19]. Combinations of estramustine phosphate and vinblastin as well as combining endocrine therapy with chemotherapy are reserved for the 15 to 20% of patients who do not respond to first-line endocrine treatment [19]. These treatments are discussed in depth in the next chapter by H. Scher.

Luteotrophic Hormone Releasing Hormone Agonists

The introduction, a decade ago, of the luteotrophic hormone releasing hormone agonist (LHRH-A), which offers a complete and reversible medical castration, found instant response in patients and physicians alike. The slow release depot preparation is now widely used. Goserelin, the most extensively studied biodegradable depot preparation, is dispersed throughout a matrix of lactide glycolide copolymer, the basic ingredient of surgical catgut; this provides a medical castration lasting for one month. LHRH-A has no reported side-effects besides the physiological surge of T at the time of the first injection. The expected side-effects are, of course, lack of libido, impotence and hot flushes.

Landmark phase III trials confirmed the equivalence of subjective and objective response rates and time to treatment failure between LHRH-A and surgical castration or DES [20,21].

The reversibility of LHRH-A treatment offers the patient a safe option to wait for the treatment results, enjoy his possible remission and switch to surgical castration for convenience if required. The physiological side-effect of the initial injection provoking a T surge may cause a transient worsening of signs and symptoms in patients with a heavy metastatic burden. The reported incidence of this side-effect concerns around 5% of all patients. A true clinical complication is rare but it is prudent to give these patients anti-androgens before or concomitant with the first LHRH-A depot injection for the first week [22].

Anti-Androgens

The anti-androgens are a class of drugs that block the androgen receptors in the presence of normal or even elevated levels of dihydrotestosterone (DHT). There are two types of anti-androgens: steroidal anti-androgens with progestational activity and non-steroidal or pure agents that are devoid of any hormonal effect.

The progestational anti-androgens have a dual mode of action. They block the androgen receptors in the prostatic tissue but also inhibit the release of luteotrophic hormone (LH) by their antigonadotrophic action. Cyproterone acetate (CPA) is widely used as a steroidal anti-androgen in Europe while other progestational, anti-androgenic compounds are used in the United States and Japan. CPA was used to treat, among other diseases, hypersexuality in men and it is no surprise that the side-effects of the usual oral dose of 100 to 300 mg/day include loss of potency as testosterone castration levels are recorded with these dosages. In an EORTC study, CPA 250 mg/day produced identical survival results to 3 mg/day of DES with a lower risk of cardiovascular toxicity [23]. The clinical use of CPA, besides primary monotherapy, includes prevention of a flare-up of LHRH analogue therapy, a quality that it shares with the non-steroidal anti-androgens, and reduction of hot flushes after orchidectomy or LHRH-A treatment [24]. It is difficult to compare the efficacy of CPA against the non-steroidal anti-androgens. The side-effects of the widely used anti-androgens are presented in Table 4 and one notices immediately that effective CPA treatment is apt to cause impo-

Table 4. Side-effects of anti-androgens in the reported daily dosage

Side-effect	Cyproterone acetate	Flutamide	Nilutamide	Casodex
Gynaecomastia	+	+	+	+
Liver toxicity	+	+	±	-
Nausea/vomiting	-	+	+	-
Diarrhoea	-	+	-	-
Visual problems	-	-	+	-
Lung toxicity	-	-	+	-
Effects on libido	++	±	±	±
Cardiovascular effects	+	-	-	-
Alcohol intolerance	-	-	+	-

tence while potency can be maintained with different doses of anti-androgen treatment using flutamide or casodex. We await the results of the EORTC trial 30892 in patients with metastatic prostatic cancer and good prognostic factors that compares 300 mg/day of CPA versus 750 mg/day of flutamide. The ultimate aim is to define the least toxic treatment for these patients with emphasis on their quality of life. The bottom line is that CPA has been demonstrated in quite a number of phase II and phase III trials to be effective and accepted as monotherapy in advanced prostatic cancer. In contrast to flutamide, combination therapy with CPA concurrently with bilateral orchidectomy or LHRH agonist could not be demonstrated to improve time to progression or overall survival [25].

The non-steroidal compounds block androgens also at the receptors of the hypothalamic-pituitary level, activating a compensatory increase in LH and resulting in increased serum testosterone levels. The 3 most widely used anti-androgens are flutamide, nilutamide and casodex, all structurally related. The appeal of these agents as monotherapy is that they can prevent impotence in sexually active patients. The stabilisation and even a slight increase in serum testosterone values might be responsible for the conservation of libido and potency. The increase noted in a number of patients may explain the high serum oestradiol levels which are converted by peripheral aromatisation and which cause gynaecomastia [26]. The difference between these drugs lies in their toxicity profiles (see Table 4) and their pharmacokinetics. The recommended daily dosages are: flutamide 250 mg 3x/day, nilutamide 300

mg daily and casodex 50 to 150 mg daily.

The biological and clinical properties of flutamide were reported in 1972 [27]. Subsequent open phase II studies reported up to 87.5% of favourable responses in patients with advanced prostatic cancer; a mean survival of 50 months in a second study was reported in patients who had objective responses [28,29]. These favourable responses did not come out in phase III trials where flutamide was compared to stilboestrol or estramustine [30,31]. In an ongoing EORTC trial flutamide is being compared to CPA. No randomised studies with nilutamide as monotherapy have been performed as yet. Despite this lack of evidence, a number of urologists use either drug as monotherapy at initial diagnosis with emphasis on the desire of the patient to keep his potency.

Casodex, which was developed in 1981, with high anti-androgenic activity and a half-life of 7 days, has now been used in over 3,000 patients for periods of up to 6 years [32]. The first reports in phase II studies evaluating casodex at 50 mg showed objective and symptomatic response [33], but phase III studies comparing 50 mg casodex to bilateral orchidectomy showed a slight inferiority in terms of time to progression and survival [34]. In regard to these results, a new trial comparing 100 and 150 mg of casodex showed an identical safety profile as the 50 mg dose but a symptomatic improvement that was as good as bilateral orchidectomy. We have to wait for the final analysis to conclude that casodex 150 mg daily identifies its benefits and risks as monotherapy. Most clinical interest in the non-steroidal anti-androgens has been focussed on their role in combination with bilateral orchidectomy or LHRH agonists to achieve maximal androgen blockade (MAB).

Maximal Androgen Blockade

Anti-androgens are able to compete with the adrenal derived DHT for the occupation of the androgen receptors in prostatic tissue after the elimination of testicular androgens by surgical or medical castration. The first phase II studies reported by Bracci on a combination with CPA and by Labrie et al. on a combination with flutamide created and still create controversy regarding the final clinical benefit of MAB treatment [35,36]. The controversy is now coming to an end thanks to a series of workshops organised by the American Cancer Society, the European Organisation for Research and Treatment of Cancer and the International Prostate Health Council, in which all randomised trials with an MAB treatment arm were analysed and prepared for a meta-analysis [25]. The last results reported show substantial advantages in progression-free survival rates in the studies involving flutamide and nilutamide and increased survival rates have been reported in several studies [13,38]. The interpretation of these results as an advantage to the patients is being analysed in ongoing studies which address the true meaning of progression-free survival with regard to quality of life, while the benefit of survival seems only substantial in patients with minimal disease. A large prospective trial organised by the South West Oncology Group (SWOG) comparing bilateral orchidectomy and placebo to bilateral orchidectomy and flutamide will allow a statistical analysis of the trends regarding the importance of prognostic factors such as minimal disease. It is remarkable that none of the trials with CPA as the anti-androgen in combination treatment has shown any difference in progression-free or overall survival. Follow-up analysis of the results of a number of ongoing trials might also give support to the MAB concept or contradict it. Another reason for caution is, of course, the reports on the flutamide withdrawal syndrome which seems to be confirmed by a number of different studies [39]. While awaiting the final conclusion, we recommend MAB treatment where LHRH agonists are used, at least in the first 14 days to avoid flare-up, especially in patients with extensive tumour burden and in patients who prefer the most efficacious hormonal treatment with disregard of impotence.

Alternative Combination Treatments

Favourable results have been reported with other combination schemes. A promising combination seems supplementation of DES 0.1 mg with a progestational anti-androgen [40]. Intermittent androgen blockade or withdrawal has been studied by several groups but these concepts have not been tested in phase III trials. The rationale is that the temporary interruption of the androgen blockade might repopulate the tumour burden with more androgen-sensitive cells.

Chemotherapy can be added to initial hormonal treatment in patients with poor prognostic factors. EORTC study 30893 is comparing orchidectomy with and without mitomycin C while the National Prostatic Cancer Project (NPCP) showed an advantage over buserelin, an LHRH agonist, by adding methotrexate to castration [41].

Patient's Choice of Treatment

Sensibilisation training of general practitioners and more informed involvement of the patient and his family can lead to an improved exchange of information with the treating urologist regarding the indications and expectations of proposed treatment. The current gap in our knowledge of the prognostic factors that predict disease outcome, the difficulty in measuring response and progression, the quality-of-life considerations and the lack of effective treatment for metastatic hormone-independent prostate cancer make it very difficult to aim at truly informed consent on the part of the patient and at his ability to evaluate various primary hormonal treatment proposals. What are the data? In a review of the mean survival in a number of consecutive EORTC trials in patients with metastatic prostatic cancer, it can be noticed that the median survival has steadily increased over the last 15 years. It is tempting to attribute this finding to improvements in treatment, but unfortunately we have reason to believe that better patient selection and better prognostic factors may be involved. Still the sad truth is that the mean survival in our last EORTC trial 30853, analysed for patients with metastatic disease, was 27 months for those treated with bilateral orchidectomy and 34 months for those treated with MAB treatment. We also see that, in contrast to the population mortality statistics, about 80% of our patients die specifically of prostate cancer and not of related diseases. Here, the bottom line is that metastatic prostatic cancer is definitely a lethal disease in which the discussion must be focussed on extended time to progression-free and overall survival and quality of life is of prime importance.

The question is how to reconcile the best treatment for response and survival with the best treatment for the patient. Here, the statistical analysis of the phase III trials is subordinate to a choice of primary endocrine treatment, tailored to the options and the choice of the individual patient. The usual questions that will be asked are, not necessarily in the same order: what exactly is wrong with me, am I going to die from this disease, do I need treatment if I don't have symptoms, will the treatment be affecting my body and my way of life and, in the very last place, how much time and money do I need to spend on the treatment? It is quite simple to demonstrate to the patient that no other treatment besides endocrine treatment produces subjective and objective responses at that rate and that he has to make a choice. The first choice is between surgical and medical castration. In view of the fact that the results of endocrine treatment including castration are unpredictable, most patients accepting castration prefer the reversible medical castration for the first 6 months. It is a matter of common sense and it gives them a certain guarantee that the sacrifice of their male physiology and sexuality is worthwhile. The great majority again prefer the clean medical castration by injection of LHRH-agonist depot preparations.

The next question is if an anti-androgen should be added to the medical castration. Again, if there is a great tumour burden or serious clinical discomfort caused by metastatic pain, it is wise to prime the patient first with anti-androgens, followed by the initial LHRH-A depot injections. Exceptions to this general rule are excruciating pain due to metastasis or impending collapse of a vertebral body visualised by imaging techniques at the time of diagnosis. This would be an indication for immediate bilateral orchidectomy or parenteral injection of oestrogens. The latter could be a polyoestradiol phosphate or an estramustine phosphate preparation. The next question is then, based on the available knowledge, whether the anti-androgens should be continued or not. So far, the meta-analysis shows only a minor trend towards increased overall survival for the MAB treatment, but important studies in which progression-free survival based on strict response and progression criteria was incorporated, show a definite advantage in progression-free survival for the combination. Again, without statistical confirmation, common sense shows clearly that patients with poor prognostic factors have no time to enjoy these differences since their mean survival is only 18 months. Based on the available data, one would think that patients with good prognostic factors or even moderate prognostic factors will profit most from the combination. The introduction of PSA as the most important marker for prostatic disease and quite reliable in disease monitoring provided us with a practical motive to continue MAB treatment after the first two weeks. A decrease to normal levels indicates an excellent response and predicts a good prognosis [42]. Here, if no toxicity from the added medication occurs, one can stick to the old dictum that one should never change a winning team.

We face a more delicate problem with the patient who wants to preserve his sexuality as an important part of his quality of life. We have no scientific proof that monotherapy with non-steroidal anti-androgens is as effective as surgical or medical castration. Still, there is enough evidence from the phase II studies and the ongoing phase III trials with casodex in the 150 mg/day dose that results come close to castration, again confirmed by the percentage of patients with PSA normalisation after initial treatment. The available data support the clinician in his choice to use the non-steroidal anti-androgens with strict monitoring of the disease parameters to start a monotherapy with these compounds. We have followed a number of patients treated with flutamide and recently casodex, the latter in a randomised trial, to predict a promising response. Some of these responses have been stable for up to 5 years. An annoying side-effect, however, is the development of breast tenderness and gynaecomastia. The patient treated with anti-androgen monotherapy is warned that an insufficient response after 3 months will warrant the addition of surgical or medical castration to the regimen. We consider this an early sign of incomplete response to endocrine treatment and we prefer to perform a bilateral orchidectomy in these cases since the normal development of treatment will go towards additional chemotherapy. Complete surgical castration is abandoned in favour of a bilateral subcapsular or subepididymal orchidectomy.

It is evident that patients with cardiovascular side-effects are excluded from treatment with oestrogenic or progestational agents.

If the patient is confronted with the different options at the time of initial diagnosis and is fully aware that the first 3 months of treatment will test the response of the tumour to the chosen treatment, a flexible situation for treatment adaptation is created. It is then much easier to apply the MAB treatment in two steps or even select surgical castration if endocrine treatment shows no results and the loss of sexuality looks secondary to the problem of survival.

The bottom line is that adequate endocrine treatment means at least a surgical or a medical castration, ideally complemented with an anti-androgen. The selection criteria to choose treatment tailored to the outcome expected by the patient are presented in Table 5. There is, of course, still room for an option of no treatment outside the ongoing trials. We recommend in these cases that no biopsy be made if no treatment is intended. We recommend that such patients be closely watched, with, among other procedures, PSA determination in the follow-up.

Adjuvant Treatment

Adjuvant treatment has to be considered in patients with special pathology or poor prognostic factors. Long acting oral morphine preparations and non-steroidal anti-inflammatory drugs should be given if no dramatic pain relief is obtained with endocrine treatment in patients with painful bone metastasis. Solitary bone metastasis that causes pain should be considered for radiation treatment already at the initial diagnosis. Further development of bone seeking radiopharmaceuticals and diphosphonate compounds is in progress. The threat of spinal cord compression has to be recognised in all patients and immediate treatment with steroids and radiation therapy and, in selected patients, surgical decompression should be part of the overall treatment of patients with metastatic disease.

Again, long responding patients and patients with poor prognostic factors should be considered for initial combination treatment of endocrine therapy and chemotherapy. Unfortunately, few chemotherapeutic drugs have consistently shown lasting clinical responses which make them suitable for inclusion in the daily practice of first-line treatment to patients with metastatic prostate cancer. Mitomycin C, high-dose epirubicin and methotrexate have brought about remissions, and so have liarozole, suramin and somatostatin analogues in patients with progression. All of these drugs are still in the realm of clinical research where as much attention should be paid to the drug regimen as to the status of the patient subjected to the trial. A more recent form of clinical research is the use of neo-adjuvant endocrine therapy in patients with localised disease. There are clinical data to support the concept that the primary tumour responds more frequently and progresses less frequently than distant metastasis, especially bone metastasis [43].

The search for early prostate cancer stimulated by the clinical development of transrectal ultrasound and later by serum PSA determination,

Table 5. Selection of primary endocrine treatment as a choice of the patient

Patient's status	Possible choice
Cardiovascular risk	Avoid oestrogenic and progestagenic compounds
Prefer to keep sexuality	Non-steroid anti-androgens
Fear of surgical castration	
Body image	Subcapsular/subepididymal bilateral orchiectomy
Physiology	Anti-androgens
Lack of response	LHRH agonists
Prefer efficacy	MAB treatment
Prefer low cost, no bother	Surgical castration

shifted the initial treatment towards the probability of cure by radical prostatectomy or radiotherapy. This shift in treatment led to renewed interest in the old concept of downgrading and downstaging the primary tumour by giving neo-adjuvant endocrine treatment for a few months before radical prostatectomy or concomitantly with radical radiotherapy. A great number of conflicting reports added to the confusion but the interest of even the more sceptical observer was stirred by reports that about 10% of patients treated with MAB before surgery had no tumour found in the pathology specimen despite step sectioning of the entire prostate [44]. This prompted other groups to launch a randomised trial, organised by the European Study Group on Neo-Adjuvant Treatment of Prostate Cancer [45].

Conclusions and Future Directions

Controversies about primary hormonal treatment are the net result of our incomplete understanding of the prognostic factors at initial diagnosis and after treatment. The lack of randomised trials of sufficient size to stratify these factors and identify the proper cohorts of responding patients makes it impossible to select the one and only first-line endocrine treatment. Here lies precisely the point that prostate cancer, a disease of the older generation, despite its continuum as a tumour, presents itself as many different diseases in different subsets of patients. Defining the right treatment, offering disease-free survival advantages for the right cancer in the right patient, will be our main goal for the year 2000. If we keep in mind that we are discussing palliative treatment instead of cure, we know we should always direct our therapeutic intention towards the patient's quality of life as seen by himself. Disease

monitoring by measuring serum PSA and hormones related to the symptoms and the objective measurable disease of the patients can be used to adjust a chosen treatment. We look forward to the results of a number of randomised trials to support the concept that treating this disease in a multihormonal environment where many factors stimulate or inhibit cancer growth can lead to personalised treatment for each man affected by this disease.

Monotherapy with anti-androgens, a combination treatment by definition, still offers a legitimate hope that refinement of the blockade by the development of new compounds or by adding finasteride could push MAB treatment to further total androgen blockade specifically for the prostate, as was recently reported from a pilot study. A randomised, prospective trial, organised by the International Prostate Health Council, will address this issue.

Refining the primary endocrine treatment given at early stages of the disease will improve the subjective and objective clinical results but does not resolve the basic problem of the hormone-independent cancer cells that are present in most tumours. Novel cytotoxic drugs, immunomodulatory drugs, monoclonal antibodies directed against the cells and new drug delivery systems are needed to switch from palliative treatment to treatment with curative intent. We hope, although we cannot be optimistic, for a shattering breakthrough in this field as well as in the chemoprevention of prostate cancer which is now definitively launched by the initiation of a trial by the National Cancer Institute. We do hope that these and other research efforts will culminate in success for our patients by the year 2000. Until then, we have to include the concept of quality of life in all our evaluations and develop the tools that allow us to define and monitor any treatment that will give more life to years than years to life [46].

REFERENCES

1   Denis LJ: Controversies in the management of localised and metastatic prostatic cancer. Eur J Cancer 1991 (27):333-341
2   Hermanek P and Sobin LH: TNM Classification of Malignant Tumors, ed 4, rev 2. Springer Verlag, Berlin 1992.
3   Smith PH, Bono A, Calais da Silva F, Debruyne F, Denis L, Robinson M, Sylvester R, Armitage TH and the EORTC Urological Group: Some limitations of the radioisotope bone scan in patients with metastatic prostatic cancer: A sub-analysis of EORTC trial 30853. Cancer 1990 (66):3-10
4   Denis L: Staging and prognosis of prostate cancer. Eur Urol 1993 (24):13-19
5   Soloway MS, Hardeman SW, Hickey DP, Todd BB, Soloway SM, Moinuddin M, Memphis TN: Simple grading system for bone scans correlates with survival for patients with stage D2 prostatic cancer (abstract). J Urol 1987 (138):359
6   Cooper EH, Armitage TG, Robinson MRG, Newling DWW, Richards BR, Smith PH, Denis L and Sylvester R: Prostatic specific antigen and the prediction of prognosis in metastatic prostatic cancer. Cancer 1990 (66):1025-1028
7   Huggins C, Stevens RE and Hodges CV: Studies of prostatic cancer II. The effects of castration on advanced carcinoma of the prostate gland. Arch Surgery 1941 (43):209-228
8   Denis L and Mahler C: Prostatic cancer: An overview. Rev Oncol 1990 (3):665-677
9   Veterans Administrative Cooperative Urological Research Group: The effects of treatment on survival of patients with cancer of the prostate. Surg Gynecol Obstet 1967 (124):1011-1017
10   Bailar JC and Byar DP: Estrogen treatment for cancer of the prostate: Early results with 3 doses of diethylstilbestrol and placebo. Cancer 1970 (26):257-261
11   Adolfsson J, Ronstrom L, Carstensten J, Lowhagen T and Hedlund PO: The natural course of low grade, non-metastatic prostate carcinoma. Br J Urol 1990 (65):611-614
12   Johansson J, Adams H and Anderson S: Natural history of localised prostatic cancer. Lancet 1989 (1):799-803
13   Denis LJ, Whelan P, Carneiro de Moura JL, Newling D, Bono A, De Pauw M, Sylvester R and Members of the EORTC GU Group and EORTC Data Center: Goserelin acetate and flutamide versus bilateral orchiectomy: A phase III EORTC trial (30853). Urology 1993 (42):119-129
14   Cassileth BR, Soloway MS, Vogelzang NJ et al: Patients' choice of treatment in stage D prostate cancer. Urology 1989 (33):57-62
15   Glenn JF: Subepididymal orchiectomy: The acceptable alternative. J Urol 1990 (144):942-944.
16   Robinson MRG: Complete androgen blockade: The EORTC experience comparing orchidectomy versus orchidectomy plus cyproterone acetate versus low-dose stilbestrol in the treatment of metastatic carcinoma of the prostate. In: Murphy GP, Khoury S, Küss R, Chatelain C, Denis L (eds) Prostate

Cancer Part A: Research, Endocrine Treatment and Histopathology. AR Liss, New York 1987, pp 383-390
17   Aro J: Cardiovascular and all-cause mortality in prostatic cancer patients treated with estrogens or orchiectomy as compared to the standard population. The Prostate 1991 (18):131-137
18   Benson R and Hartley-Asp B: Mechanisms of action and clinical uses of estramustine. Cancer Investigation 1990 (8):375-380
19   Seidman AD, Scher HI, Petrylak D, Dershaw DD and Curley T: Estramustine and vinblastine: Use of prostate specific antigen as a clinical trial end point for hormone refractory prostatic cancer. J Urol 1992 (147):931-934
20   Kaisary AV, Tyrrell CJ, Peeling WB and Griffiths K: Comparison of LHRH analogue (Zoladex) with orchiectomy in patients with metastatic prostatic carcinoma. Br J Urol 1991 (67):502-508
21   Citrin DL, Resnick MI, Guinan P, Al-Bussam N, Scott M, Gau TC and Kennealey GT: A comparison of Zoladex R and DES in the treatment of advanced prostate cancer: Results of a randomized multicenter trial. The Prostate 1991 (18):139-146
22   Schulze H and Senge T: Influence of different types of antiandrogens on luteinizing hormone-releasing hormone analogue-induced testosterone surge in patients with metastatic carcinoma of the prostate. J Urol 1990 (144):934-941
23   de Voogt HJ: The position of cyproterone acetate (CPA), a steroidal anti-androgen, in the treatment of prostate cancer. The Prostate 1992 (4):91-95
24   Jansen JE: Prevention of hot flushes with cyproterone acetate (CPA). In: Murphy G, Khoury S, Chatelain C, Denis L (eds) Recent Advances in Urological Cancers: Diagnosis and Treatment. FIIS, Paris 1990, pp 70-71
25   Denis L and Murphy GP: Overview of phase III trials on combined androgen treatment in patients with metastatic prostate cancer. Cancer 1993 (72):3888-3895
26   Mahler C and Denis L: Clinical profile of a new non steroidal anti-androgen. J Steroid Biochem Mol Biol 1990 (37):921-924
27   Neri R, Florance K, Koziol P and Van Cleave S: A biological profile of a non steroidal anti-androgen Sch 13521. Endocrinology 1972 (91):427-437
28   Sogani PC, Vagaiwala MR and Whitmore WF: Experience with flutamide in patients with advanced prostatic cancer without prior endocrine therapy. Cancer 1984 (54):744-750
29   Prout GR, Keating MA, Griffin PP and Schiff SF: Long-term experience with flutamide in patients with prostatic carcinoma. Urology 1989 (34):37-45
30   Lund F and Rasmussen F: Flutamide versus stilboestrol in the management of advanced prostatic cancer. A controlled prospective study. Br J Urol 1988 (61):140-142
31   Johansson JE, Lingärdh G, Andersson SO, Zador G and Beckman KW: Clinical evaluation of flutamide and estramustine as initial treatment of metastatic carcinoma of prostate. Urology 1987 (29):55-59
32   Furr BJA, Valcaccia B, Curry B, Woodburn JR, Chesterton G and Tucker H: ICI 176;334. A novel non steroidal peripherally selective anti-androgen. J

Endocrinol 1987 (113):R7-R9

33 Tyrrell CJ: Casodex: A pure non-steroidal anti-androgen used as monotherapy in advanced prostate cancer. The Prostate 1992 (4):97-104

34 Kaisary AV: Current clinical studies with a new, non-steroidal antiandrogen Casodex (ICI 176,334). Clinical Developments in Prostate Cancer, 1993 (abstract). Satellite Symposium held at the 2nd International Congress of the Dutch Urological Association, Amsterdam, 3 November 1993

35 Bracci U: Anti-androgens in the treatment of prostatic cancer. Eur Urol 1979 (5):303-306

36 Labrie F, Dupont A and Bélanger A: A complete androgen blockade for the treatment of prostate cancer. In: de Vita VTJr, Hellman S, Rosenberg SA (eds) Important Advances in Oncology. JB Lippincott, Philadelphia 1985, pp 193-200

37 Denis L and Mettlin C: Conclusions from the American Cancer Society workshop on combined castration and androgen blockade therapy in prostate cancer, Atlanta, Georgia, September 18-20, 1989. Cancer 1990 (66):1086-1089

38 Crawford ED, Eisenberger MA, McLeod DG, Spaulding JT, Benson R, Dorr FA, Blumenstein BA, Davis MA and Goodman PJ: A controlled trial of leuprolide with and without flutamide in prostatic carcinoma. N Engl J Med 1989 (321):419-429

39 Kelly WK and Scher HI: Prostate specific antigen decline after antiandrogen withdrawal: the flutamide withdrawal syndrome. J Urol 1993 (149):607-609

40 Goldenberg S, Bruchovsky N, Rennie PS, Coppin CM and Brown EM: The use of synergistic hormonal combinations in the treatment of advanced prostatic cancer: cyproterone acetate plus mini-dose diethylstilbestrol. Proceedings of the International Symposium on Hormonal Manipulation of Cancer: Peptides, Growth Factors and New (Anti)Steroidal Agents, 1986, June 4-6, Rotterdam, The Netherlands

41 Huben PR, Murphy GP and the Investigators of the National Prostatic Cancer Project: A comparison of diethylstilboestrol or orchiectomy with buserelin and with methotrexate plus diethylstilboestrol or orchiectomy in newly diagnosed patients with clinical stage D2 cancer of the prostate. Cancer 1988 (62):1881-1887

42 Oesterling JE: Prostate specific antigen: A critical assessment of the most useful tumor marker for adenocarcinoma of the prostate. J Urol 1991 (145):907-923

43 Schröder FH: What is new in endocrine therapy of prostatic cancer ? In: Newling DWW, Jones WG (eds) Prostate Cancer and Testicular Cancer. Wiley-Liss Inc, New York 1990, pp 45-52

44 Fair WR, Aprikian A, Sogani P, Reuter V and Whitmore WF: The role of neoadjuvant hormonal manipulation in localized prostatic cancer. Cancer 1993 (71):1031-1038

45 Witjes WPJ, Horenblas S, Oosterhof GON, Schaafsma HE and Debruyne FMJ: Neoadjuvant therapy in prostate cancer - Is it of any use ? Eur Urol 1993 (24):433-437

46 Calais da Silva F, Reis E, Costa T, Denis L and Members of the Quality of Life Committee of the EORTC Genitourinary Group: Quality of life in patients with prostatic cancer. Cancer 1993 (71):1138-1142

Hormone-Independent Prostate Cancer: Management of the Disease Continuum

Howard I. Scher

Genitourinary Oncology Service, Division of Solid Tumor Oncology, Department of Medicine, Memorial Sloan-Kettering Cancer Center, 1275 York Avenue, New York, New York 10021 and Department of Medicine, Cornell University Medical College, New York, U.S.A

Neoplastic diseases of the prostate, both benign and malignant, are the result of or are associated with a sequence of genetic changes. While the sequence of these molecular events is under study, recent evidence suggests that both benign prostatic hyperplasias and malignancies of the prostate may be part of similar pathways. Currently, it is unclear if benign lesions are precursors of malignant change. The malignant spectrum also represents a continuum of disease, ranging from a clinically silent or latent form to palpable local lesions and ultimately to metastases. It is postulated that additional genetic alterations are associated with or required for further progression. In most patients these changes evolve over many years. As a result, there are many competing causes of death in addition to the tumour, particularly in elderly patients with localised lesions, and many patients die "with" as opposed to "from" the disease. Thus, a key to selecting the appropriate treatment for an individual patient, is to refine our ability to define the biological and clinical potential of a tumour.

It has been recognised for many years that prostate cancers are under the influence of androgen. The effects are mediated directly on epithelial cells or secondarily through the stromal components of the gland by stimulation of growth factor production. Growth factors produced in the stroma, for example, may stimulate epithelial cells in a paracrine fashion. However, as tumours evolve locally to become clinically palpable, a parallel change occurs rendering some of the cells capable of growing independently of androgen stimulation. Consequently, androgen ablation results in the regression and death of some, but not all, of the epithelial cells present in a tumour. This has been shown in both animal models, and studies of clinically localised (T2-3) prostatic cancers treated with androgen ablation followed by radical prostatectomy. Whether this is the result of an intrinsic insensitivity of the epithelial cells to androgen ablation, an adaptive effect to the castrate milieu, or the result of continued stimulatory effects from the surrounding stroma is not understood. These observations explain why androgen ablation is not curative for patients with metastatic disease, and that to favourably impact on survival requires the use of treatments that are directed against androgen-independent cells.

An additional feature of prostatic neoplasms is the interactions between the stromal and epithelial components of the gland. The former can serve a permissive role, i.e., support growth factor action, or a directive one, i.e., induce a permanent phenotypic change in the responding epithelial cell. In the development of prostatic cancers, both mechanisms are contributory. Recent work by Chung et al. suggests that the extracellular matrix may irreversibly affect the differentiation of prostate epithelial cells and render non-tumorigenic cells tumorigenic. These stromal effects are organ specific. For example, fibroblasts from the extracellular matrix derived from the bone or from the prostate facilitate prostatic epithelial cell growth, while fibroblasts from the liver will not [1]. It is also likely that the phenotype of the tumour cells in different sites may not be the same, as they may be under distinctly different influences in different sites, and will not respond uniformly to treatment. Tumour heterogeneity also contributes to the spectrum of responses seen in the primary and metastatic sites.

Patterns of Progression

Prostate cancers that have progressed following hormonal therapy are, for the majority of patients, predictable in their course. Clinically, progression can manifest itself in several ways. In some cases there is asymptomatic yet incremental increase in a biochemical parameter such as prostate-specific antigen; new areas of increased uptake - indicative of new bony lesions - on radionuclide scan, an increase in pain or, less frequently, progression in soft-tissue disease. In other cases, a parallel increase in PSA and in soft-tissue disease is documented. A distinct pattern of rapid soft-tissue progression without a rise in PSA, or a rise in PSA that is disproportionately low relative to the "tumour burden" occurs in approximately 15-20% of patients. This may represent a "small cell" conversion which requires a unique therapeutic approach with combination chemotherapy (*vide infra*). These patterns of progression suggest that there are inherent biological differences between tumours in different sites (Table 1).

The therapeutic programme for hormone-refractory prostatic cancer at Memorial Sloan-Kettering Cancer Center is based on the following hypotheses: 1) tumours that proliferate in the absence of androgen, i.e., androgen-resistant lesions, are not the same as the tumours that were present at the time of the original diagnosis and must be characterised separately; and 2) the ability of prostate cancers to metastasise and proliferate in selected sites

Table 1. Hormone-refractory disease: patterns of progression

Measurable disease:	Adenocarcinomatous differentiation
	Neuroendocrine differentiation
Osseous disease only	
Elevation in PSA	

Adapted from Scher and Cordon-Cardo [3]

such as bone, is the result of the favourable trophic influences of the microenvironment that renders the tumour cell relatively resistant to treatment. We have developed this theme in the clinic by repeating biopsies of hormone-independent lesions, and by recommending treatment on the basis of the predominant metastatic pattern in an individual patient.

The Initial Evaluation

Recognising that there is no curative therapy available for hormone-refractory disease, and that the therapeutic goals are largely palliative, it is important to learn to anticipate the disease and treat potentially problematic areas before they become symptomatic. This can be critical for areas that can adversely affect quality of life. In patients with prostatic cancer the most debilitating symptoms relate to pain from bony metastases, spinal cord compression and/or progressive primary disease which can result in ureteral obstruction and renal failure, or urinary retention if left untreated. In other cases a generalised debilitation syndrome develops that can result in fatiguability, anorexia and weight loss. The latter results in what has been described by many as a patient "fading away". Our approach at the initial consultation involves a full re-evaluation with particular attention to several issues: symptoms, documentation of the anorchid state, restaging procedures to fully assess the pattern of progression, and optimising medications.

A careful history can provide important information with regard to selection of treatment. A simple question of "What is the major symptom that you are experiencing" that we can try to alleviate - pain, urinary frequency, weakness, fatigue - can provide great insight. In some cases, fatique is the result of sleep deprivation from nocturia. Careful attention to what medications a patient is taking and with what frequency they are taking them is also important. It is surprising how many patients have inadequately controlled pain syndromes, regardless of the aetiology. For example, patients who are awakened by pain, are in general receiving inadequate dosages of analgesics and have significant pain. Many are afraid to take "narcotics" for fear of addiction or dependence, and few have been appropriately instructed on the need to maintain chronic steady-state levels of these medications by repetitive dosing. Even fewer receive adequate information on regulation of bowel function in conjunction with narcotic analgesics. In some cases, patients will say they have "minimal pain", when in fact they have compensated for a severe pain syndrome by becoming increasingly sedentary. Others will describe severe "movement-related pain", with minimal pain at rest. Often we will ask a patient to rate their pain on a scale of 1 to 10. Those who reply that the pain intensity is 5 or more are, as a rule, affected to the point where the pain level has significantly compromised their functional status. In our experience, careful attention to and patient education on the use of analgesics is of tremendous clinical benefit. Once this aspect of treatment has been resolved, the evaluation can proceed to define the aetiology of the pain, which, in the population with prostatic cancer, is not always related to metastatic disease. Other symptoms that are specifically addressed at the initial visit include fatiguability, diet, weight loss, urination pattern and frequency, bowel function, and symptoms that might suggest neurological compromise.

In addition to the routine aspects of the physical examination, careful notation of the findings on rectal examination that might clinically indicate local progression should be documented. A careful examination of the spine and nervous system is also important and any signs or symptoms suggestive of cranial nerve, spinal cord, or cauda equina compromise must be vigorously pursued.

The laboratory evaluation is also standardised. For patients who have not undergone surgical castration, a testosterone level is checked to insure that the patient is truly anorchid. In some cases where progressive disease is documented, physicians will advise discontinuation of hormonal therapies such as gonadotropin hormone releasing hormone (GnRH) analogues. Cost considerations undoubtedly enter into the recommendation to discontinue treatment in some cases. This can result in a rise in testosterone levels which can accelerate the disease and shorten survival. In these situations, reinstitution of androgen ablative therapy can result in palliation, albeit short-lived in most cases, while the evaluation continues. Further, if a GnRH analogue is to be restarted, pre-treatment with an anti-androgen is important to block the flare reaction. A complete blood count is done to insure that the patient is not anaemic or has other signs of marrow compromise. An assessment of hepatic and renal function is also performed. In some cases an elevation of the serum transaminases can occur as the result of anti-androgen therapy, and does not necessarily reflect metastatic disease. Hepatic dysfunction has been shown to reduce PSA clearance, leading to higher values than might be anticipated based on the extent of disease. If an elevation in serum creatinine is documented and renal compromise is confirmed radiographically, consideration can be given to the placement of ureteral stents, nephrostomy tubes, a transurethral resection, or palliative radiation therapy. Finally, prostate-specific markers - prostate-specific antigen and acid phosphatase - are also checked and compared to previous examinations to assess the tempo of the disease.

A bone scan is performed to evaluate the progression of the disease and to identify areas that may potentially become problematic. For example, an intense lesion in the thoracic spinal cord should be evaluated with plain films and, if clinically indicated, magnetic resonance imaging or myelography. This area of the spinal cord frequently remains clinically silent despite significant spinal cord compromise. Those areas with compromise should be treated with external beam radiation therapy whether or not they are symptomatic. It is also important to recognise that these syndromes can develop quickly, and that just because a patient had a normal neurological evaluation 3 months prior to the current evaluation, does not insure that epidural disease has not developed in the interval. In general, our policy has been to obtain plain films of areas that have shown significant progression or that are symptomatic. If plain films show a lytic component, external beam radiation should be recommended sooner rather than later. While it may be difficult to prove that this approach is more beneficial in terms of prolongation of survival, the chance of a durable response to radiation therapy is increased when the tumour is small and less painful. Further, prevention of spinal collapse or spinal cord compromise would seem desirable.

Our evaluation also includes a CT scan to insure that there is no soft-tissue disease, as reliance on PSA determinations alone can be misleading. For example, it is known that tumours dedifferentiate with time and there is the possibility of conversion to a more anaplastic histology. In some cases, significant pelvic, retroperitoneal or visceral disease may be observed on the scan despite low values of PSA or acid phosphatase. Those with progressive soft-tissue disease, or residual disease in the primary are advised to have a repeat biopsy performed to better define the pathologic phenotype of the progression. In most cases, however, the pattern of progression is either an asymptomatic rise in prostate-specific antigen, or symptomatic progression in bone. Our clinical trials are based on these patterns of progression: bone only, biochemical or soft-tissue.

Separation of Trials Based on Patterns of Progression

Table 2 identifies distinct populations of patients with hormone-refractory disease who can be considered for treatment. The distinct endpoints of clinical investigations are also included.

Bone Only Disease

A unique therapeutic approach for bone metastases is required for several reasons. Firstly, after androgen ablation, only 25% of bone lesions actually improve by scan compared to 82% of soft-tissue lesions. Secondly, at 2-year, progression in bone is 4 times more

Table 2. Chemotherapy trial designs

Patient population:	"PSA" only
	Measurable disease
	Initial therapy (poor prognosis patients)
	Chemohormonal therapy
Endpoints:	Objective tumour regression in measurable disease
	Decline in PSA
	Palliation (pain relief)
	Time to progression
	Survival

frequent than soft-tissue progression, suggesting that the disease is not eliminated after androgen ablation in the first place [2]. Thirdly, an analysis of patients treated at MSKCC on phase II measurable-disease protocols showed that 80% first progressed in bone despite a response in soft tissue, again suggesting that bone is relatively resistant to treatment. Overall, our experience has been that response in bony sites manifested by a decrease in prostate-specific antigen (PSA), an improvement in a bone scan or plain radiograph is rare. These clinical observations provide further evidence that the bone microenvironment renders cells relatively resistant to both hormonal and chemotherapy. Indeed, several growth factors that are specifically mitogenic for prostate epithelial cells have been isolated from bone.

PSA Elevations

Rising levels of PSA in the setting of castrate levels occur in over 90% of cases of patients who are progressing after primary therapy. When documented on serial determinations, it is indicative of tumour growth, as shown by the fact that clinical symptoms such as pain, ureteral obstruction, or spinal cord compromise will develop in most patients after a median of 3-4 months. Thus, in our view, progressive elevations in PSA justify a change in treatment in most patients. Further, it was on this basis that we, and others, began to investigate posttherapy PSA changes as an outcome measure for clinical trials. Additional study on the prognostic significance of the rate of rise in PSA is ongoing. It has been shown, for example, that the doubling time for some localised prostatic cancers can exceed 2 or more years. If this were the case in an elderly patient with asymptomatic hormone-refractory disease, one might consider a period of observation without treatment. For the majority of patients with hormone-refractory disease, however, median survivals rarely exceed one year, which justifies therapeutic intervention.

Measurable Disease

The "gold standard" for evaluating chemotherapeutic agents in phase II trials is to treat a cohort of patients with bidimensionally measurable disease parameters in whom response can be assessed. Previously at MSKCC, we restricted entry on clinical protocols to patients who met these criteria, approximately 10% of the population with hormone-refractory disease. Using this approach, 10 single-agent trials have been completed with partial responses in 0-24% of cases, with an overall median survival of 6.3 months [3]. This suggested the need for a change in strategy.

Clinical Trial Designs

Post-Therapy Changes in PSA

Recognising the difficulties in evaluating response or progression in bone, and considering that over 90% of patients with progressive hormone-refractory disease have elevations in PSA, we developed the following methodology to "standardise" the use of PSA change as a clinical trial outcome measure. First, for entry on study we require a documented rise in PSA of 50% or more on two successive occasions. This was derived from a phase II trial in patients with measurable disease where this degree of elevation antedated measurable disease progression in all cases. Further, we have empirically chosen a minimum PSA value of 40 ng/dl (> 20 ng/ml if the prostate has been removed) for entry. As a measure of response, we felt it important to define both a degree of decline and a duration for which it was maintained. Thus we initially proposed an >80% decrease from the baseline value (degree of decline) for a minimum of 3 biweekly determinations (duration) as a "partial response" (Table 3). This was derived from the observed corre-

lation between an 80% decline from baseline and measurable disease response in patients treated with androgen ablation [4].

More recently, however, we completed a prognostic factor analysis of pre and post-therapy variables for survival in patients with hormone-refractory disease treated with different therapies. Patients were followed until death or censored if still alive. In univariate analysis, a pre-treatment haemoglobin ≥ 13.0 g/dl (p=0.001), normal alkaline phosphatase (p=0.0004), lactate dehydrogenase ≤ 230 (p<0.001) and Karnofsky performance status ≥ 80 (p=0.002) were associated with a good prognosis. Considering post-therapy parameters, and using a landmark of 8 weeks for the outcome measure, a comparison of the survival distributions of patients who showed a 50% decline from baseline vs. those who did not, showed a median not reached vs. 8.1 months, respectively (logrank test, p=0.0002). These observations were validated on an independent data set of patients treated at the Norwegian Radium Hospital in Oslo, Norway. Of interest was that the survival distributions of the patients treated in the United States and in Norway were similar, and that the patients with measurable disease and evaluable (bone only) disease had comparable median survivals [5].

The results of this type of trial must be interpreted cautiously for several reasons. First, some of the chemotherapeutic agents administered inhibit the release of PSA from tumour cells independent of the effect on cell kill. Fluctuations in PSA levels can occur without treatment. However, these rarely exceed ± 20% from baseline. In addition, as a tumour differentiates, PSA levels may increase, which may reflect a beneficial effect of therapy. Finally, it is well recognised that PSA expression in a tumour is heterogeneous, raising the

Table 3. Proposed response criteria using PSA as an endpoint

Complete Response (CR):	**Normalisation** of the PSA for 3 successive evaluations
Partial Response (PR):	Decline of PSA value by ≥ **80% or** ≥ **80%** (without normalisation), for 3 successive evaluations
Stabilisation (STAB):	Patients who do not meet the criteria for PR or PROG for at least 90 days
Progression (PROG):	**Three** consecutive increases in PSA, to **> 50% above baseline**

Table 4. Proposed strategy for evaluating new agents in prostatic cancer based on post-therapy changes in PSA

STEP

1   Trial using PSA decline as endpoint → no effect → discard

                    EFFECT

2   Clinical trial in measurable disease → no effect → discard

                    EFFECT

3   Phase III trial in hormone-refractory disease

                    EXPERIMENTAL THERAPY
                              VS.
                    BEST SUPPORTIVE CARE

4   Phase III trial in "poor-risk" patients with hormone-naive disease

                    EXPERIMENTAL THERAPY
                              VS.
                    STANDARD HORMONAL THERAPY

Modified after Scher and Cordon-Cardo [3]

possibility that a treatment may have an effect only on the cells which actually secrete PSA, or that an effect on the non-PSA secreting cells may be missed.

We have therefore developed this strategy as part of a sequence of trials (Table 4). First, a cohort of patients with elevated PSA levels are treated. If no "responses" are observed, the agent is discarded. If "response" is observed in a predefined proportion, a group of patients with measurable disease are enrolled. If antitumour activity is confirmed (step II), the agent(s) can be tested in a large scale phase III trial using survival as the endpoint (step III and IV). Ultimately, if the observation that response based on PSA declines correlates with the results based on a measurable disease population, and considering that the survival distributions between measurable and evaluable disease patients are similar, it may be possible to eliminate step II in this sequence. At present, however, the observation that a 50% decline from baseline at 8 weeks based on 3 biweekly determinations needs confirmation before it can be used as a definitive measure of efficacy.

Therapeutic Approaches Based on Pattern of Progression

Bone Only Disease: Radiolabelled Diphosphonates

In most patients the metastatic spread to the skeleton is diffuse, which makes durable palliation of pain difficult despite control of selected sites with external-beam radiation therapy. Bone seeking radiopharmaceuticals take advantage of the chemical properties of the carrier molecule to selectively deliver radiation therapy to tumour bearing regions and have been used therapeutically to treat painful lesions. It is, however, important to recognise that palliation of pain can occur without a direct antitumour effect. A similar dissociation has been observed with low-dose corticosteroids [6], cold diphosphonates, and the bone resorption inhibitor gallium nitrate [7], and may result from an inhibitory effect on the release of local mediators such as prostaglandins or growth factors, or from a direct toxic effect on bone osteoclasts.

An alternative hypothesis is that there may be sufficient tumour cell kill at the site of deposition of the isotope to produce pain palliation without affecting measured PSA values. Thus, to assess these effects of these agents in the clinic, the endpoint of change in pain intensity must be considered independent of the effect on the tumour. This can be very difficult and must include a consideration of who is doing the pain assessment, i.e., the patient, the nurse, the physician or a spouse, and the frequency with which it is assessed. Analgesic consumption must also be considered. Ideally, one would aim for a reduction in pain with a reduction in the consumption of analgesics, as a reduction in pain with an increase in analgesics would not represent a beneficial effect of treatment. An assessment of antitumour effects can be performed using sequential changes in PSA. This is the approach we have adopted at MSKCC where parallel evaluations of pain intensity, measured on a twice daily basis, daily analgesic consumption in morphine equivalents, and weekly PSA changes are evaluated. Bone seeking radioisotopes that have been used in the clinic include derivatives of 32P, 89Yt-EDTA and 89-strontium which have the disadvantage that they are dosed empirically because they do not emit gamma energies that allow imaging. Although palliation has been observed, in most cases myelosuppression has been dose limiting. 186-ReHEDP [Rhenium-186 (Tin) hydroxy ethylidene diphosphonate] and Sm-153-EDTMP [Samarium-153 phosphonic acid [1,2-ethyanediyl bis [nitrilobis (methylene)]] tetrakis-monohydrate] are metal diphosphonates with radioactive moieties that emit gamma energies that provide images similar to technetium-99 MDP scans, and short-range energies that permit therapy. Rhenium-186 HEDP localises to the inner cortical layer of the osteoblast (H.R. Maxon, University of Cincinnati, personal communication), the primary change induced by prostatic cancer in the skeleton is an osteoblastic reaction. At the University of Cincinnati, a phase II trial of patients with pain secondary to prostatic cancer in the skeleton showed palliation in 16 of 20 (75%, 95% confidence limits 62-98%) [8]. At MSKCC, entry on protocol required at least one painful lesion in an area that had not received prior external beam radiation therapy with no restrictions on the extent of prior radiation therapy or chemotherapy. Patients were treated with 35 mCi every 8 weeks for up to 4 administrations. Daily pain intensity and pain relief were measured on 100 mm visual analogue scales which are components of the Memorial Pain Assessment Card (MPAC) [9]. These scales were completed on a daily basis and analgesic consumption normalised to morphine equivalents.

Of the first 27 patients treated, of whom 24 required narcotics, a decrease in pain intensity was noted in 18 (67%, 95% confidence limits 49-85%). The maximal benefit was observed by week 2 and maintained through week 5. No change in analgesic consumption was noted. A dissociation between the pain response and antitumour activity was observed as antitumour activity (> 80% decline in PSA from baseline) was observed in only 2 cases (7%, 95% confidence limits 0-17%). Toxicities were acceptable. A second trial investigating escalated administered activities is ongoing. Preliminary data show that injections of 80 mCi are well tolerated, and that the maximal tolerated dose has not been reached. Similar results have been observed using 153-Sm-EDTMP.

Second-Line Hormonal Therapy

Several groups have evaluated second-line hormonal therapies using PSA changes as the endpoint. However, the criteria for a favourable outcome with respect to the degree of PSA decline and the duration for which it is maintained, have not been standardised. For example, with the use of stilphosterol declines ranging from 44-93% from baseline in 13 of 29 cases were reported (45%, 95% confidence 27-63%), while ketoconazole produced a mean decrease of 49% of 4 months' duration in 12 of 15 cases (80%, 95% confidence 60-100%), and flutamide resulted in declines of 40% or greater in 7 of 24 cases (29%, 95% confidence 11-47%), while this is an agent not considered efficacious as second-line treatment (reviewed in [3]). Thus, the results of these trials must be interpreted cautiously.

Assessing the true response to second-line hormonal therapies in patients with prostatic cancer is hampered by the heterogeneity of the patient population treated and the response criteria used. Patient variables include factors such as whether the patient had a prior orchiectomy or not, extent and duration of response to prior endocrine therapy, pretherapy serum and, probably of greater importance, intratumoral hormonal levels. In addition, many reports include "stable disease" in a response category, which is difficult to assess, particularly when the disease is limited to osseous sites. Further, most studies were completed prior to the availability of PSA determinations. Nevertheless, some patients do benefit from a second trial of hormones as shown by Tannock et al., who noted palliation of symptoms in 33% of cases treated with low-dose prednisone [6].

The Flutamide Withdrawal Syndrome

Apart from the responses observed by the addition of a second hormonal agent, we have observed sustained declines in serum PSA ranging from 37-89% in 3 sequential patients after discontinuation of the anti-androgen flutamide for a median of 3 months. One had a normalisation of the alkaline and acid phosphatase. This was associated with clinical improvement in the one patient with symptoms. Similar declines in PSA have been observed in 6 subsequent patients who also had flutamide withdrawn. All had demonstrated a 2-8 fold increase in PSA on hormonal therapy prior to discontinuation of the anti-androgen [10]. While the mechanism responsible for this observation has not been defined, it would seem reasonable to give a trial of "flutamide discontinuation" prior to the initiation of a second hormone or chemotherapy. Furthermore, these data further emphasise the cautious interpretation of post-therapy declines in PSA, and the need to document progression prior to enrollment in a clinical trial.

Mechanism-Based Therapy in Patients with Rising PSA Levels or Measurable Disease

Microtubule inhibition

Estramustine phosphate (EMP) is oestrogen with a phosphate group at the C17 position and nor-nitrogen mustard in position 3 (Fig. 1). Although patients treated with the compound develop oestrogen-like effects, cytotoxicity is not related to steroid action, and the compound does not show alklyating agent effects since the carbamate bond is resistant to cleavage in vivo. The cytotoxic effects are due to the disruption of microtubules and inhibition of microtubule assembly through binding to microtubule assembly proteins. Tissue culture studies have shown EMP to be an antimitotic agent, blocking tumour cell division in metaphase. The intracellular target(s) are distinct from those of vinca alkaloids such as vinblastine and vincristine, which exert their antimitotic effects via binding to tubulin. It also targets the nuclear matrix, suggesting the possibility of synergy with topoisomerase inhibitors (Ken Pienta, personal communication).

In a recently completed multi-institutional study of 42 patients with hormone-refractory disease treated with estramustine (14 mg/kg/day) alone, 21% (95% confidence interval 9-34%) of patients had a greater than 50% reduction in PSA, and 31% had subjective pain relief using the MPAC scale [11]. As a phase II trial at M.D. Anderson showed activity for vinblastine administered by continuous infusion, and based on the reported synergy between estramustine and vinblastine against prostatic cancer cell lines in vitro, we evaluated the combination of the two agents in patients with hormone-refractory disease using post-therapy changes in PSA as the endpoint. Using a schedule of 10 mg/kg/day p.o. of estramustine and 4 mg/m^2 of vinblastine weekly for 6 weeks followed by 2 weeks rest, 13 of 24 patients (54%, 95% confidence 34-74%) responded using PSA criteria (>50% decline), while 2 of 5 patients with measurable disease responded [12]. Two independent trials at M.D. Anderson and Fox Chase Cancer Center reported declines in PSA in 11 of 22, and 17 of 37 cases, with measurable disease response in 3 of 7, and 3

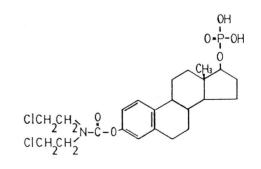

Fig. 1. Structure of estramustine phosphate

of 7 cases, respectively. In aggregate, 43% (35/82, 95% confidence interval 32-53%) of patients showed a >50% reduction in PSA, with measurable disease response in 42% (8/19, 95% confidence limits 20-64%). Phase III trials are planned. Additional studies with the combination of estramustine and oral etoposide are ongoing, with encouraging preliminary results (Dr. Ken Pienta, personal communication).

Growth factor inhibition

The more rapid proliferation of metastatic bone vs. primary prostate lesions and the observation that the separation of prostatic epithelial cells from their surrounding stroma inhibits epithelial cell proliferation, are part of an increasing body of evidence that autocrine and paracrine production of growth factors contributes to prostate cancer cell growth *in vivo*. These factors act at the external cell surface by binding and activating specific transmembrane glycoprotein receptors. Several classes of growth factors, including the epidermal growth factor (EGF)/transforming growth factor alpha (TGFα), basic and acidic fibroblast growth factor, transforming growth factor beta (TGFß), insulin growth factor (IGF), platelet derived growth factor (PDGF), and nerve growth factor (NGF) have been isolated from conditioned media of human-derived prostate cancer cell lines, extracts from prostatic tissues or identified in cut sections of human tumours by immunohistochemical techniques. Based on *in vitro* studies showing that inhibition of growth factor action can inhibit prostate cell growth, several groups have undertaken clinical trials aimed at blocking growth factor action *in vivo*.

The first agent brought to clinical trial based on its putative growth factor inhibitory effecs was suramin, a polyanionic compound that inhibits the binding and the mitogenic effects of a number of polypeptide growth factors (Fig. 2). This agent, however, is not specific and has a number of other effects including: inhibition of glycosaminoglycan synthesis, membrane-associated ion pumps, protein kinase C, glycolysis, and inhibition of the metastatic process through effects on cell motility [13]. The rationale for testing suramin in prostatic cancer was based on the antitumour activity against prostatic cancer cell lines *in vitro* and *in vivo*; the inhibitory effects on the mitogenic effects of the specific growth factors produced by prostatic epithelial cells and their surrounding stroma, and the effects of suramin on adrenal steroidogenesis. As a result, all patients treated with suramin receive hydrocortisone concomitantly [14].

A variety of dosing regimens have been evaluated, most used a continuous infusion regimen where the drug was continued until a target concentration of 280-300 µg/ml was reached. The latter was based on a suggestion that dose limiting toxicities, of which a severe peripheral neuropathy was the most feared, were related to peak suramin concentrations. Other dose-limiting toxicities including a polyradiculopathy, myelopathy, renal insufficiency, coagulopathy, and vortex keratopathy, only increased patient and physician anxiety of the compound. As a result, early trials required intense plasma concentration monitoring, making administration of the compound impractical and complex.

In spite of the concerns about the compound, if one summarises results from several centres,

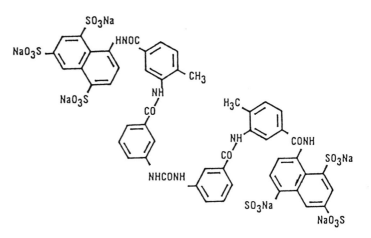

Fig. 2. Structure of suramin

35% (35/111, 95% confidence interval 20-42%) of patients with measurable disease have shown a greater than 50% reduction in size, while 44% (71/166, 95% confidence interval 34-54%) showed a greater than 50% decline in PSA. In addition, several groups have observed responses that last beyond one year, making suramin one of the most active agents against hormone refractory disease. As a result, intensive study has gone into simplifying the administration of the compound and more recently, however, it has been shown that the therapeutic index can be improved using outpatient bolus doses without plasma concentration monitoring, and the significance of the 300 µg/ml upper limit has been questioned. In addition, the drug has shown to be synergistic with tumour necrosis factor, adriamcyin, and more recently, radiation therapy, and combination trials are underway.

"Traditional" chemotherapeutic agents

While no single agent or combination regimen has been shown to improve the survival of patients in a phase III randomised trial, it must be remembered that many of the reported results using "standard" agents were based on response criteria developed prior to the availability of PSA. In addition, many drugs were tested in a patient population with an inherently poor prognosis, in part due to a general phobia of chemotherapy. It was therefore not surprising that the reported results were poor. This was recognised by the investigators of the National Prostatic Cancer Project who developed separate protocols for patients who had received and who had not received extensive radiation therapy. As most chemotherapeutic agents have a steep dose rate/response curve, inadequate dosing virtually guarantees failure. Currently, as patients and physicians recognise the significance of steadily increasing PSA levels, more patients with a good performance status who have not received extensive radiation therapy and chemotherapy are entering clinical trials. The results have been interesting in that some of the agents believed to be inactive based on prior experience, are showing significant antitumour activity that is clearly worthy of further study.

For example, high-dose cyclophosphamide (4.5 g/m^2 I.V. q 2 w) with granulocyte-macrophage colony stimulating factor (GM-CSF) support produced a >80% decrease in PSA in 4 of 10 patients (40%) [15]. In contrast, a lower dose schedule (1 g/m^2 I.V. q 3 w) had an objective response proportion of 4% in 151 evaluable cases (95% confidence interval 1-8%) using the criteria developed by the NPCP prior to the use of PSA. The reported response proportions to adriamycin range from 0-84%, depending on the cases selected for treatment and the response criteria used. More recently, doxorubicin was combined with 5-fluorouracil and in a separate trial with ketoconazole. In the first trial, objective responses (>50% reduction in PSA or >50% reduction in measurable disease) were observed in 61% of cases (11 of 18, 95% confidence 39-84%), while the second showed biochemical response in 57%, with measurable disease regression in 7 of 11 cases (64%, 95% confidence 35-92%) [16]. Taken together, these results suggest that prostatic cancers may not be as refractory to treatment as previously believed.

Small-Cell Tumours and Neuroendocrine Differentiation: Rapid Soft-Tissue Progression with Low PSA Levels

Cells with neuroendocrine features can be found in the majority of primary prostate tumours on careful histological examination. The significance of these cells was not fully appreciated until recently. The cells are generally interspersed throughout the gland, occur independently of grade or pathological stage, and can secrete polypeptide hormones such as calcitonin, serotonin, glucagon, ACTH, somatostatin, parathyroid hormone and thyroid stimulating hormone. Under light microscopy, the most frequent change is focal neuroendocrine differentiation in a conventional adenocarcinoma, although in some cases pure small-cell changes are apparent. Clinically, this variant should be suspected when there is rapidly progressive disease, visceral metastases and disproportionately low PSA levels relative to the total tumour burden. In our experience, it can be identified in approximately 15% of cases and is important to be recognised because these tumours are sensitive to regimens used to treat small-cell tumours of the bronchus (such as etoposide and cisplatin or cyclophosphamide, adriamycin and vincristine), regimens that are generally not used for the more conventional adenocarcinomas.

Future Directions

Antibodies to Cell Surface Antigens: Immunophenotyping

It is recognised that prostatic cancers become more aggressive over time, but few studies have focussed on serial pathological changes over different periods. Most treatment decisions are based on the histology obtained at the time of diagnosis. Recently, for example, we have shown that the pattern of expression of the epidermal growth factor receptor changes from a predominantly basal pattern to a more homogeneous pattern as the tumour goes from a hormone-naive primary to a hormone-refractory metastatic lesion. This would suggest that strategies aimed at inhibiting the epidermal growth factor receptor would be of therapeutic importance. These studies are planned. In addition, a number of monoclonal antibodies to prostatic epithelial cells are under investigation. While most have been evaluated as potential imaging agents, by attaching different radioactive ligands there is the potential for use of these agents for therapy. For example, several antibodies have been developed using prostate cancer cell lines as immunogens, and among these PR92 (DU-145), F77-129 (PC-3) and CYT 356 (LNCaP) are in clinical trial. The results of imaging studies show the heterogeneity of prostatic cancers *in vivo*. Thus, prior to use of these agents, direct biopsy characterisation of the tumour to be treated will be important [3].

Differentiation Therapy: Retinoids

Interest in the retinoids stems from the observation that all trans-retinoic acid has: direct cytotoxicity observed *in vitro*, differentiation effects, inhibitory effects on tumour development in animal models, and has been shown to down-regulate TGFα expression in germ cell tumour cell lines. These agents bind to nuclear receptors that act as transcription factors and that serve to regulate specific differentiation

programmes. Clinical trials in human prostatic cancer have recently been initiated.

Conclusions

Hormone-refractory disease is not as resistant as previously believed. Several treatments, shown in the laboratory to have inhibitory effects on human prostate cancer cell lines, have proved to benefit a proportion of patients. Clinical trials of these agents suggest several promising leads for further study. These include the putative growth factor inhibitor suramin, and the combination of estramustine and vinblastine. A key to benefit with these agents is their use in patients who are less symptomatic, and who received less prior therapy. In short, patients who are not endstage. The availability of serial PSA determinations allows the identification of treatment efficacy early, so that ineffective therapies can be discontinued and the patient spared needless toxicities.

In addition, it has become apparent that hormone-refractory disease is not one disease, but represents a spectrum of disease with different clinical manifestations in individual patients. The importance of characterising the tumour in an individual is shown by the range of pathological findings observed with respect to growth factor expression and monoclonal antibody phenotyping. In addition, a proportion of patients show a significant neuroendocrine component, which requires a unique therapeutic approach. In these cases, an aggressive chemotherapeutic approach, which is not effective for patients with the more typical adenocarciomas, is of benefit. Of equal importance is that with careful attention to the patterns of progression in an individual patient, the debilitating symptoms of the disease can be averted for many patients. This alone can improve quality of life, a critical factor for a disease which is not curable with currently available therapies.

Acknowledgement

Supported by CA-05826 and CM-01-57732 from the National Institutes of Health and a grant from Mallinckrodt, Inc, St. Louis, Mo., and The Michael Wolff Fund for Prostate Cancer.

REFERENCES

1   Gleave ME, Hsieh JT, von Eschenbach AC and Chung LW K: Prostate and bone fibroblasts induce human prostate cancer growth in vivo: implications for bidirectional tumor-stromal cell interaction in prostate carcinoma growth and metastasis. J Urol 1992 (147):1151-1159

2   Goldenberg SL, Bruchovsky N, Rennie PS and Coppin CM: The combination of cyproterone acetate and low dose diethylstilbestrol in the treatment of advanced prostatic carcinoma. J Urol 1988 (138):1460-1465

3   Scher HI and Cordon-Cardo C: Current and future therapeutic strategies in metastatic hormonal resistant prostate cancer: therapy based on phenotype. Problems in Urology 1992

4   Miller JI, Ahmann FR, Drach GW, Emerson SS and Bottaccini MR: Clinical usefulness of serum prostate specific antigen after hormonal therapy of metastatic prostate cancer. J Urol 1992 (147):956-961

5   Kelly WK, Scher HI, Mazumdar M and Vlamis V: Prostate specific antigen (PSA) as a measure of disease outcome in hormone refractory stage D2 prostate cancer. J Clin Oncol 1993 (11):607-615

6   Tannock I, Gospodarowicz M, Meakin W, Panzarella T, Stewart L and Rider W: Treatment of metastatic prostatic cancer with low-dose prednisone: evaluation of pain and quality of life as pragmatic indices of response. J Clin Oncol 1989 (7):590-597

7   Scher HI, Curley T, Geller N, Dershaw D, Chan E, Nisselbaum J, Alcock N, Hollander P and Yagoda A: Gallium nitrate in prostatic cancer: evaluation of antitumor activity and effects on bone turnover. Cancer Treat Rep 1987 (71):887-891

8   Maxon HR, Schroder LE, Thomas SR, Hertzberg VS, Deutsch EA, Scher HI, Samaratunga RC, Libson KF, Williams CC, Moulton JS and Schneider HJ: 186-Re(Sn)-HEDP for the treatment of painful osseous metastases: initial clinical experience in 20 patients with hormone resistant prostatic cancer. Radiology 1990 (176):155-159

9   Fishman B, Pasternak S, Wallenstein SL et al: The Memorial Pain Assessment Card: a valid instrument for the evaluation of cancer pain. Cancer 1987 (60):1151-1158

10 Kelly WK and Scher HI: Prostate specific antigen decline after antiandrogen withdrawal. J Urol 1993 (149):607-609

11 Yagoda A, Smith JA, Soloway MS, Tomera K, Seidmon EJ, Olsson C and Wajsman Z: Phase II study of estramustine phosphate in advanced hormone refractory prostatic cancer with increasing prostate specific antigen levels. J Urol 1991 (145):384A (Abstract)

12 Seidman AD, Scher HI, Petrylak D, Dershaw DD and Curley T: Estramustine and vinblastine: use of prostate specific antigen as a clinical trial end point for hormone refractory prostatic cancer. J Urol 1992 (147):931-934

13 Scher HI: Suramin: here to stay? JNCI 1993 (85):594-597

14 Myers, C, Cooper M, Stein C, LaRocca R, Walther MM, Weiss G, Choyke P, Dawson N, Steinberg S, Uhrich MM, Cassidy J, Kohler DR, Trepel J and Linehan WM: Suramin: a novel growth factor antagonist with activity in hormone-refractory metastatic prostate cancer. J Clin Oncol 1992 (10):881-889

15 Smith DC, Vogelzang NJ, Goldberg HL, Gockerman JP, Winer EP and Trump DL: High-dose cyclophosphamide (CTX) with granulocyte-macrophage-colony stimulating factor (GM-CSF) in hormone-refractory prostatic carcinoma. Proc Am Soc Clin Oncol 1992 (11):213

16 Logothetis CJ, Dexeus F, Chong CDK, Sella A and Finn L: Cytotoxic chemotherapy for hormone-refractory metastatic prostate cancer. In: Johnson DE, Logothetis CJ and von Eschenbach AC (eds) Systemic Therapy for Genitourinary Cancers. Year Book Medical Publishers, Chicago 1992 pp 234-238